Pathological Child Psychiatry and the Medicalization of Childhood

D0076504

Currently, it is common practice among the child psychiatric establishment to prescribe powerful and potentially addictive drugs to children who have emotional or behavioural problems. *Pathological Child Psychiatry and the Medicalization of Childhood* is a strong challenge to this way of thinking.

Sami Timimi uses a wide variety of sources, including his personal experiences, to highlight the role of culture, beliefs, science, social hierarchy and power in shaping our understanding of childhood problems and how to deal with them. He urges professionals who work with children to question their assumptions in a manner that will enable them to access a greater variety of potentially helpful therapeutic frameworks.

Since the 1960s, psychiatry has had to learn to accommodate critical analysis of its beliefs and methods. The legitimacy of its core assumptions continues to be questioned. Now child psychiatry too must engage with such a debate if it wishes to develop into a genuinely democratic and inclusive profession. *Pathological Child Psychiatry and the Medicalization of Childhood* will be of great interest to professionals and trainees in psychiatry and child psychiatry, social work, family therapy and other psychotherapies for children and adolescents.

Sami Timimi is a consultant child and adolescent psychiatrist who works full time in the National Health Service in Lincolnshire. This is his first book. He has previously published many articles in academic journals on a variety of topics including cross-cultural psychiatry, psychotherapy and eating disorders.

Pathological Child Psychiatry and the Medicalization of Childhood

Sami Timimi

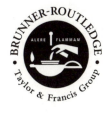

LIBRARY
FRANKLIN PIERCE COLLEGE
RINDGE, NH 03461

First published 2002 by Brunner-Routledge
27 Church Road, Hove, East Sussex BN3 2FA

Simultaneously published in the USA and Canada
by Brunner-Routledge
29 West 35th Street, New York, NY 10001

Brunner-Routledge is an imprint of the Taylor and Francis Group

© 2002 Sami Timimi

Typeset in Times by Keystroke,
Jacaranda Lodge, Wolverhampton
Printed and bound in Great Britain by
TJ International Ltd, Padstow, Cornwall
Paperback cover design by Amanda Barragry

All rights reserved. No part of this book may be reprinted or
reproduced or utilized in any form or by any electronic,
mechanical, or other means, now known or hereafter
invented, including photocopying and recording, or in any
information storage or retrieval system, without permission in
writing from the publishers.

British Library Cataloguing in Publication Data
A catalogue record for this book is available from the British Library

Library of Congress Cataloging in Publication Data
A catalogue record for this book has been requested

ISBN 1–58391–215–0 (hbk)
ISBN 1–58391–216–9 (pbk)

Contents

Preface

When I was doing my child psychiatry specialist training one of the consultants asked me if I wanted to help him with a research project looking at rates of attention deficit hyperactivity disorder (ADHD) in children with learning difficulties. I agreed and went off to do the groundwork, including a literature search. It was the first time I had looked in any depth at the ADHD literature. I kept reading this stuff over and over, trying to make sense of what this ADHD syndrome was meant to be medically. Surely it wasn't just children who are hyperactive and distractible, surely there was more to it. But there wasn't. I couldn't believe it, here we were clearly using a construct with very little medical meaning and with this fancy sounding name as if we were diagnosing something very sophisticated that required our specialist doctor skills to spot. I wrote up my literature search and took it back to the consultant who thanked me. I then told him about how reading this literature had raised lots of doubts concerning the medical validity of ADHD. He politely told me that I didn't understand phenomenology.

I decided to look into the ADHD literature further and, with the help of a consultant more sympathetic to my ideas, wrote a paper questioning the validity of the ADHD construct and raising concerns about how it might be (mis)used by child psychiatrists and other doctors. This consultant suggested I submit this paper to a medical journal, which I did. The reviewer's reply was astonishing. Up until this paper I had been playing the game in the same way most junior grade career doctors do. I had done my bit of research and written plenty of articles as sole or co-author. I was used to receiving replies from reviewers either rejecting or suggesting changes to a submitted manuscript. I had never received a reply like the one I received for this paper. Instead of concentrating on what the reviewer felt might be the short-comings of this paper, they attacked it in a very personal manner. Comments like 'these are old hat, redundant arguments that have long been dismissed as irrelevant' and 'the author has produced a paper written in a very unscholarly manner' and 'we gave our medical students a similar project some years ago and I'm sad to say even they managed to produce more sober and reflective essays'. I had touched a raw nerve. My article was blasphemous. I went to ADHD conferences; the issues I had written about were not even mentioned let alone discussed. Yet when I presented my paper to several groups of other professionals I found a very receptive audience.

I became a consultant. Freed from the mentorship system of training whereby clinical work is supervised in a hit-or-miss way by hit-or-miss consultants, I was able to begin to let go of some aspects of my training and develop new ways of working. I was helped enormously by working in a part of London with a high percentage of ethnic minority children and families. I had to re-open my mind to working with different values and belief systems.

One day, after doing a presentation on cross-culture working with health advocates, a clinical psychologist came up to me and said 'I'm not sure I heard you right, did you say you're a psychiatrist?' I said 'yes'. She looked at me in disbelief 'I find that hard to believe. How have you survived in your profession with beliefs like that?' I said 'with great difficulty'. She said 'I can imagine'. My mind was made up, the only way that these views may see the light of day in a place where some doctors might read them would be in a book.

Acknowledgements

To the individuals that have had the biggest influence on the way I practice, my stepdaughter, Michelle, and my wife, Kitty, my son, Lewis, and my daughter, Zoe. To my mother and father for raising me and protecting me. To my grandmother, Daphne, who looked after me for a year. To the rest of my family and my friends. To my therapist who helped me grow up. A huge thank you to all the clients I have had the privilege of working with and who have taught me so much. A special thanks to those families who gave permission for their stories to be included in this book.

To the many professional colleagues who have influenced the way I practice including Eia Asen, Ann Miller, Inga Britt-Krause, Rabia Malik, Zethu Makatini, Percy Aggett, Begum Miatra, John Gordon and all the therapists on the Asian family counselling service at the Marlborough clinic in London. I would like to thank my wife, Kitty, for her help with typing this book and to Kitty again, my mum, Al Wadsworth, and my secretary, Heather, for their help in the final stages of preparing this manuscript.

Chapter 1

On becoming a child and adolescent psychiatrist: a personal account

I found my psychiatric training a very confusing business. There were so many different theoretical frameworks which often produced very different accounts, conclusions and courses of action about the same clinical picture, and so many professionals with passionately held strong beliefs in the truthfulness of their approach and the incorrectness of others. Perhaps I was particularly sensitive to these seemingly irreconcilable differences as a result of my earlier experience of growing up in two very different cultures. I lived mainly in Iraq until I was 14 years old (my father being Iraqi). When I was 14, and because of the political problems in Iraq, my older brother and I came to live in England. We stayed with relatives in this country (my mother being English) until the rest of my family joined us a year later. The contrast between adolescent culture in England where I came to live and the one I left behind in Iraq couldn't have been greater. I had to change so many of my beliefs and attitudes to try and fit in with my new peer group. For whatever reasons, my experience of psychiatric training brought back familiar echoes of the confusing feelings I had as a 14-year-old trying to get my head round a kind of culture shock. Feeling strongly about one approach one day, then rejecting it the next. Trying to square circles, trying to work out how this theory would fit with that theory, how this approach would fit with that approach. Having this nagging doubt about my abilities, about not fitting in, about playing roles and pretending to believe things I didn't believe. In the back of my mind a constant worry that the theories I was following were somehow not connecting with the clients I was supposed to be helping. Was this my insecurity, my clients not playing ball or something to do with the theories?

My first experience of psychiatry was as a fourth-year medical student in Scotland. As part of our assessment for this section of our training we had to interview four psychiatric in-patients, write up the interview and submit this together with some sort of formulation outlining the relevant features from the history we had taken and our provisional diagnosis. I became interested in the stories that the patients were telling me about their lives. Already I had found the approach we were being taught (which was to concentrate on collecting signs and symptoms and analysing the answers as if they were medical entities with minimal interest in the content of the answers) limiting and oppressive. I remember following the protocol at my first few interviews and getting a good pass mark for my write up. However, I found that the story of my third patient gave me a lot to think about. She had a diagnosis of schizophrenia and had been an in-patient in the hospital for many years. Despite her clearly delusional thinking I could not help but feel that her story made some sort of sense. I can only remember a few brief snapshots now of this story but I recall that she was infertile, she had had a long marriage and her husband had then died. She was religious and spoke about god gifting people with immaculate conceptions. She claimed to have had many such immaculate conceptions since her husband had died and that she had given birth to many hundreds of what she called water babies who were growing up, unseen to other people, in a river near a power station. After talking to her I went to the medical school library to look for a book which might help me make more sense of this story. After leafing through a number of fairly standard psychiatric texts I came across Dr Laing's book, *The Divided Self*. I borrowed this and read it from cover to cover. I then used this book extensively in my writing up of this particular case. I wrote a long formulation, which concentrated a lot more than the previous cases, on the story of this patient and the possible meanings her story may have. At that time I was not aware that Dr Laing was considered anti-mainstream psychiatry and so was disappointed when, having put all that effort in, I was failed on this essay. As a consequence I had to do another interview with a different patient using the standard formula in order to pass. It was my first introduction to the dictatorship of the medical model in psychiatry and the lack of respect given to alternative viewpoints.

After a gruelling and depressing year as a house officer I started my first job in psychiatry, in Scotland in August 1989. It was immediately apparent that psychiatry is, in some fundamental way, different to the rest of medicine. On my first day as a psychiatrist I attended my first psychiatric ward round. It was very different to the medical and surgical ward rounds I had got used to. For a start there were fewer patients and we spent much longer with each patient. The ward round took place in one room (as opposed to crowding round a patient's bed) where the relevant professionals sat discussing the patient. At the end of each discussion, the patient would be brought into this room full of people and the consultant psychiatrist would ask him/her a few questions. The patient would then leave and decisions (which seemed to be mainly about medication) would be made. The hierarchy, with the consultant at the top making all those decisions that were considered important, was very clear. That feeling that there was not much interest in the stories that the patients had to tell, came back to me. The ward was busy, the work stressful and emotionally loaded (with the standard advice to deny the emotional impact by keeping your distance from the patients, a very 'us and them' set up), and nobody seemed to have time to spend with the patients. I remember one patient who was seeing a clinical psychologist on a weekly basis telling me that he didn't agree with what the psychologist was saying but he really liked going to his sessions because the psychologist seemed to be showing an interest and made time to talk with him. I found this first experience of psychiatry particularly frustrating. It seemed to centre on medication. The one time I remember being openly praised by the consultant I worked for was when I made a suggestion concerning medication which she agreed with. Furthermore, having regular contact with the patients, my impression was that the cocktails of medication the patients were on did not seem to be making any real difference, certainly not as far as many of the patients were concerned. It was also my first exposure to the great divide between mental-health professionals and their clients. Psychiatrists, nurses, social workers and others frequently let off steam by 'bitching' about the patients – talking in derogatory ways about them behind their back. Face to face they would completely change. There was, for me, an uncomfortable dishonesty about this, 'nurse Smith I think you're talking about me behind my back', 'no, that's just your paranoia, your illness playing tricks on you'.

It was during this first job that I started attending psychotherapy supervision sessions run by a consultant psychotherapist. I was really taken by this and got into reading psychotherapy books, in particular psychoanalytic ones. I felt there was a huge contrast between the approach I was expected to take on the in-patient ward and the approach being taken in the psychotherapy supervision sessions. Here each supervision session would concentrate on one meeting of one therapist with one patient. The content of that one meeting would be analysed in the minutest detail with an emphasis on the meaning of the client's behaviour and speech. Medication was hardly ever mentioned. Even though the meanings being constructed were, I now believe, primarily those of the professionals, at this time in my career I found this approach a breath of fresh air and an approach that seemed to me to be more humane, even if it was particularly labour intensive. I then took on my first psychotherapy patient who was also simultaneously being seen in psychiatric out-patients by one of the consultant psychiatrists. In psychiatric out-patients she had a diagnosis, was receiving medication and presumably having very different conversations to those she was having in therapy with myself. In my sessions the diagnosis was unimportant. The emphasis was on my and my supervisor's construction of meaning as it developed in the context of her relationship with myself in the sessions, even though this peculiar relationship was only occurring for one hour once a week. As in true psychoanalytic style I was not providing any advice or answering any questions that she may have put to me. I found myself wondering what sense this patient was making of these two very different experiences, one with me and one in the out-patients, with two professionals who were both psychiatrists.

In May 1990 I came to work in London. My first impression of the psychiatric institution I started working in was a positive one. Here was a more community-orientated approach than the one I was used to in Scotland. The consultants seemed to be interested in psychological approaches in addition to medication. But, after a few months in my new job I was to be disappointed. I approached one of the consultants, who up until then I had respected for his ideas and opinions concerning a community approach to treating psychiatrically ill patients, for help with a patient I had just assessed. The consultant began showing off his knowledge of the phenomenology (psychiatric symptoms) of this acutely disturbed patient. He asked me lots of questions and then spoke about this patient, pointing out to me a lot of the theoretical fine details concerning this client's symptoms, in front of this patient as if the patient wasn't in the room. It was another sobering experience of how the stories that the patients have to tell are not viewed with respect and given any importance. What, it seems, is more important in mental-health circles, are the stories the professionals have to tell about the stories the patients are telling (and who cares what sense they make of this). I recall how excited this consultant became in his efforts to share his knowledge with me and how in that excitement it mattered little to him that the patient we were talking about was sitting in the room and being completely excluded from a conversation full of technical jargon (jargon designed, presumably, to keep clients on the outside). I began to realize that this sort of community psychiatry was the psychiatry I had got used to in Scotland with a slightly different spin.

My interest in psychoanalysis continued after my move to London and I regularly attended psychotherapy supervision seminars. The seminars themselves were often as peculiar as the psychotherapy sessions. As soon as you walked in the door of the consultant psychotherapist's room you felt yourself entering a world completely separate from the rest of the hospital. The patients we focussed on had histories not that dissimilar to the other patients I was seeing with my psychiatry hat on. Indeed, many of them were also being seen in psychiatric out-patients and/or had been in-patients in the hospital. Yet we spoke about them with a completely different language and set of ideas. The approach to helping was very different to the medical psychiatric approach and I repeatedly failed to see how one connected to the other or what sense patients made of these diverse cultural experiences, where different meanings were being given to their life problems. The psychotherapy consultant at this first hospital that I worked at in London appeared to me to be a very serious man who was always deep in thought. I can't remember him ever smiling or laughing at anything and soon I found myself carrying this sense of deep seriousness into psychotherapy sessions with patients. One common feature of both the psychiatric and the psychoanalytic approach seemed to be an emphasis on pathology and what was wrong and the seriousness of what was wrong.

In my next job at a hospital just outside London, one of my supervising consultants was a likable and creative consultant who had the habit of doodling during ward rounds. Sometimes he appeared not to be listening to what people were saying, however, by the end of the ward round he would usually have made some decisions as well as produced a few simple pencil portraits of staff members! He was the first consultant I came across with passionate beliefs that were anti-psychoanalytic. He held a strong conviction that cognitive behavioural therapy was the way forward, the answer. I ended up having many light-hearted arguments with him about the usefulness and validity of different treatment approaches. He organized a cognitive behavioural therapist to come and supervise trainees, like myself, in cognitive behavioural therapy. Here was yet another treatment approach with its own theory and beliefs. Another way of attaching meaning and significance to patient's complaints and a new professional story about patients' stories for me to learn.

During this time I also found myself returning to my medical-school interest in Dr R.D. Laing's books. I found them a refreshing escape from the confusion that the rival professional approaches left me in. I particularly liked Dr Laing's attempts to put our own profession under the microscope in the same way we put patients' lives and histories under the microscope.

Next came a 9-month stint at a therapeutic community with psychoanalytic thinking and approaches at its core. For 9 months the therapeutic effort concentrated on a small group of patients whom I saw individually and in a group on a weekly basis. The emotional contact with patients was close, intense and at times overwhelming, but seemed a lot more satisfactory to me than all my previous experiences in psychiatry up until that point. Shortly before starting this placement, I had also started my own personal therapy. Both these experiences brought home to me what a different cultural world the world of psychotherapy is to that of not only psychiatry, but also the rest of life in general. Of course prior to going into therapy I had the advantage of having already conducted psychotherapy sessions as a therapist, going to psychotherapy supervision groups and having read a lot of books about psychotherapy. Consequently, I was forearmed with a large amount of knowledge concerning what to expect from psychotherapy sessions. Yet, despite this, I found my nearly 3 years of psychotherapy a culturally peculiar experience. It took up a lot of time getting to and from my thrice-weekly sessions (not to mention a lot of money). It took a long time to get used to the unnatural and somewhat contrived set up in the consulting room, where ordinary human exchange rarely happened. Much time in sessions would be spent in silence. I also finally understood why many of my own clients insisted that my interpretations to them about the meaning of a separation (which the theory books seemed full of) were wide of the mark. None the less all that said, I did find my personal therapy a very helpful experience.

In 1992 I did my first child psychiatry job and was introduced to a totally new theoretical model and way of working. The children and adolescents I saw were viewed within the context of their families and the theorizing was now predominantly around the emotional interconnections within the patient's families. In this model diagnosis did not seem that relevant. In fact, on the diagnostic front, I got the impression that broadly speaking in child psychiatry there were only two main diagnoses, conduct disorder and emotional disorder. I was also pleased to find that medication was rarely given in this department. For the first time I had to get used to seeing and talking to families, not individuals. I enjoyed this new way of working but all the doubts about this new theoretical framework and method started emerging in the same way that they had with the other models I had been introduced to. I wondered how this new model fitted in with the other ones that I had learned and I wondered what sense the families made of our thinking and how much of it was inaccessible to them. The thinking and theorizing would often take place out of view of the families, behind one-way mirrors, in breaks in the session or before and after the session. The feedback to the family of our thinking would always be an edited version of our discussion. I felt this to be dishonest and something that put the therapists in a very privileged and powerful position over their clients. It also reinforced our own belief in our expertise and our sense that we were doing something exciting and important. Unfortunately, sometimes the sense of power that this method gave the therapists led to some crazy and disrespectful things being done to families. I remember there was a session when a family had been inadvertently double booked at the same time as an outing to a local wine bar for a member of the department who was leaving. The therapist with whom I was co-working convinced me that we could have our cake and eat it. He set a task for the family, explaining to them that we would be leaving them to do this task and watching them from behind the one-way mirror. We then left to have a drink with the others at the wine bar, returned half an hour later and made up some feedback to give to the family.

I then arrived back at the world of acute adult psychiatry, in a busy central London hospital, where many African and Caribbean (mainly second-generation) clients were admitted. I was back again with the deadening medication culture I had escaped for a short while in my previous two placements. The wards were overcrowded and understaffed. The climate of a psychiatric hierarchy that was diagnosis and medication orientated was suffocating and dehumanizing. There was little room for reflection and everyone seemed too busy to talk to clients, advocate on their behalf or give them a meaningful voice. Stereotypes were in abundance. One weekend I was the resident on-call junior psychiatrist for the hospital. Early on the Saturday, the police brought a young black man for urgent assessment. They said that they had discovered him in one of the parks behaving bizarrely and talking to himself. From the first hour after admission the (white) nurse manager began to pressure me to refer this man to a secure psychiatric unit (a locked unit for those deemed too dangerous to manage on an unlocked ward) because 'we believe he is a serious threat to our (the staff) safety'. Why? 'He is staring at us in a threatening manner.' I didn't agree with this and suggested we continue to observe him. I came to see the client regularly over the next few hours. He was not talking, refused to move and apparently continued to stare in 'a threatening manner'. I maintained that in my opinion there was no reason yet to either refer him to a secure unit or medicate him against his will. The next thing I knew, the nurse manager had contacted the consultant on call, who authorized a prescription for sedative medication to be given against this young man's wishes. Also unknown to me, the nurse manager called the police to ask for their assistance in restraining the client for the purpose of administering the medication by injection. I counted thirteen police arrive on the ward, some with riot shields, to restrain this apparently dangerous man. Following this I wrote a letter to the hospital management. I stated how concerned I was about the events of the weekend and used the phrase 'unconscious racism' in the letter. In the resulting meeting, chaired by one of the consultants, I was reprimanded for using the word 'racism' in my letter and asked to give an apology to the nurse manager. On the positive side it was also agreed that the policy of calling police to the ward needed to be reviewed.

After completing my general psychiatric training, I decided that I wanted to pursue a career in child and adolescent psychiatry. I had rejected general adult psychiatry as I didn't believe I could survive in a professional culture that was so medication centred and so lacking in its ability to engage with difference.

My experience of child mental-health services since then has, to me at least, been an extraordinary one. Different departments seem to have very different orientations in terms of the dominant theoretical model and method of working. These orientations seem not to reflect the differences in the local communities, but the preferences of the most influential consultant. My impression is that the type of service you will receive as a family, child or adolescent varies enormously from area to area as well as from therapist to therapist. A lot of the individual variation from therapist to therapist is, I think, to be expected. Personal qualities are unavoidably important in any therapeutic encounter (a subject that research does not like or know how to touch upon).

One consultant that I worked for was a fanatical believer in cognitive behavioural therapy. She refused to allow anybody in the department to use any method other than cognitive behavioural therapy (with or without medication) and had a standard method for this therapy for just about every problem. This standard approach was taught in the first few weeks of starting and you were expected to adhere to this with all children, adolescents and families that you saw. I began to appreciate the religious intensity with which some practitioners held on to their views. Working or even thinking in any other model was not allowed. In supervision sessions with her you would be told off if you used a word that she considered as belonging to a different framework. For example, I remember in one supervision session using the word 'denial'. I was told in no uncertain terms that this word was a meaningless term which had no place in that department. For the 10 months I was working in that department I felt as if I was expected to become part of a religious cult in a world surrounded by blasphemous teachings from which this consultant's mission was to cleanse us.

Rather worryingly, I came across many child and adolescent psychiatrists like the one described above who seemed very controlling with a reputation for being authoritarian and hierarchical in their attitude. I worried a lot about this and whether this was the inevitable outcome of training in child and adolescent psychiatry and perhaps of working with children and families. I often felt that these consultants had a tendency to treat their non-consultant colleagues like children. I also worried that perhaps it was the sort of personality that was attracted to working in this area and began to worry about what this said about me and whether I was destined to become another of those rather loathsome, hierarchical, controlling consultants. I also wondered whether some of this tendency may also be to do with the professional models we are taught in our training, particularly the 'how to be a good parent' models. These models tend to be rather rigid, suggest that there is one right way of being a parent, emphasize things such as calmness, positive reinforcement of good behaviour, ignoring bad behaviour and having firm rules and boundaries. Although I have found these models helpful over the years they don't seem to leave much room for alternative, perfectly successful and positive ways of parenting or for the normal imperfections that we all, as parents and people, have. Neither do they take any account of cultural variations in parenting. They also leave the therapist with a feeling of superiority; as if what they are preaching has some sort of quasi-religious truth to it. I have often had a feeling that some of the consultants I have worked with were carrying out some sort of good parenting programme on the staff, including myself. Dissent and difference of opinion is not allowed, but rather firmly and calmly ignored and the desired behaviour rewarded with a positive comment. This type of atmosphere I have found to be deadening to creativity and unbearably patronizing. Sometimes it has resulted in arguments with consultants, who leave you in no doubt that different opinions will not be tolerated and who then treat you in such a way as to leave you feeling worthless, marginalized, paranoid and isolated.

I also began to realize that child psychiatrists have a real identity problem. We are, after all, doctors and in child mental-health services end up at the top of the hierarchy, in positions of influence and power and usually as the most highly paid professionals amongst the mental-health staff in that service. Yet there are very few drugs to prescribe and all with surrounding controversy. There is a lot of disagreement about the usefulness of diagnosis or even the relevance of it. Many child psychiatrists will also practice and have had training in at least one form of psychotherapy, such as family therapy, cognitive behavioural therapy or psychodynamic psychotherapy. Therefore, for some of their time, many child psychiatrists practice the psychotherapy they are trained in and perhaps feel more like a family therapist, psychotherapist or behaviour therapist than a psychiatrist.

This insecurity has, I believe, led many child psychiatrists to push for a greater medicalization of our role. One of the consultants I trained with used a completely medical model framework for assessments and treatment and wanted me to define my professional role in those terms too. His expectations on how I should carry out my assessments were again completely different to those of the previous child psychiatry consultants I had worked for. Here I was expected to do an individual interview with each child or adolescent and then an interview with the parents. I had to concentrate on collecting signs and symptoms, take a developmental history and follow this with a physical examination of the patient, including things such as height, weight and head circumference. This was like the clerking in of newly admitted patients that I used to do as a house officer and a medical student. After I had clerked the patient in, I would then have to sit and watch this consultant repeat the interview, arrive at a diagnosis and, with every patient he saw, prescribe medication. Interest in other therapies or approaches was only in a strict medical model manner; in other words he would prescribe a certain number of, say, psychotherapy sessions and send the client to the psychotherapist. He himself would show no interest in the psychotherapy or what light it might be shedding on the situation.

My experience of child and adolescent psychotherapy was not much more encouraging. As in other fields I came across good and influential psychotherapists. What sticks in my mind, however, are things like the suitability criteria, which I often felt effectively discriminated in favour of those with a similar background to the therapist (and the surprise when a working-class client was considered to be thoughtful and articulate). There were also, what I felt to be, some crazy therapies, such as seeing a 2-year-old in psychotherapy for sibling rivalry. I did some child psychotherapy training. As part of this training I saw a 9-year-old girl twice a week for 2 years. My supervisor kept making encouraging noises about how well I was doing. In reality I felt it was a huge waste of time with little noticeable impact on the child's behaviour. My interpretations, although many may have been accurate, held little interest for her. As far as I could see she was just working hard to see how much fun she could get out of the sessions. The only thing that I felt may have been making a difference was the once-a-term meeting with girl's parents.

In my child psychiatry training I have gone from placements where I prescribed medication on no more than a handful of occasions over the course of a year, to placements where every patient received medication (out-patients and in-patients); from making grandiose interpretations focusing in on the complex emotions between family members, to ignoring all the emotions and focusing purely on the behaviour of the individual child; from focusing on early mother/infant history, to exclusively here and now forward-looking approaches.

What sense did I make of all of this? Not a lot.

Where were the connections, the cross-over points, the integration? Maybe I was too sensitive to difference. Perhaps I should have been more accepting and learned, like all well-behaved trainees, to live with this, after all living with ambivalence was one thing that my cultural upbringing had taught me.

Then came some turning points.

I read a number of articles by and met with ethnic minority therapists who, like me, did not feel any of these systems of thinking fitted with their experience of their community and their beliefs, indeed felt put down and belittled by western mental-health models and treatments.

My wife and stepdaughter have had a big influence on my thinking on mental health. From them I have learned a great deal about a completely unspoken subject in mental health and psychotherapy, that of class difference. This is an issue that we have had to struggle with given that I come from an academic, middle-class family and they come from a working-class background. At one point I was planning to do a research degree with a university on a psychoanalytic understanding of class issues in psychotherapy. I remember talking excitedly to my wife about this, after meeting with a professor who was interested in supervising me. I spoke to her about some of the ideas that the professor had discussed with me. My wife just could not relate to it. She asked me if all of this was going to take me further away from class issues rather than closer to understanding it. I remember how that conversation with her hit home. Here I was wanting to investigate and understand class issues using an academic, technical set up, language and theories which originate from a white, middle-class, intellectual body to generate a thesis that might result in a few papers to that same elite, exclusive audience. Here I was standing next to the real expert out of the two of us about to embark on a project whose language and theory only I had access to. I realized all that would come out of such a project was middle-class therapy theorizing and not working-class experience and understanding. Needless to say I decided the whole idea was a bad one and did not proceed. I still often go to my wife and stepdaughter for advice when I am stuck with some of my cases and frequently find their advice more useful than that of my professional colleagues, particularly where working-class families are concerned. I have had the experience of presenting a difficult case at a team meeting or a case presentation slot and hearing professionals come out with all sorts of fancy theories but nothing that particularly helps me know what to do next. I then go home and talk to my wife or stepdaughter who, uncluttered by fancy theories, provide me with a straightforward, intuitive, common-sense way to move forward. How come? They have not had any professional training. How come they know better sometimes?

I presented a paper to colleagues at a training institution, who were on the same child psychotherapy course as myself. The paper was about race and culture in clinical situations and its effect on transference and counter-transference feelings (that is the feelings the client has towards a therapist and the feelings a therapist has towards the client). In this paper I was trying to explain how many clients from ethnic minorities, when they come into contact with western institutions and western child psychiatrists like ourselves, often come with a fantasy (or accurate feeling) that they are being viewed as inferior, uneducated, crazy and often as in some way abusive to their children. My colleagues, it seemed, could not relate to this at all and seemed instead to want to concentrate on the gender aspects of one of the clinical examples which, I believe, they used to reinforce stereotypes that men from the developing world are invariably abusive to women. I left feeling insulted and angry, realizing that the technical language of psychoanalysis couldn't capture the feelings and experiences of those sitting on the wrong side of the cultural fence. This was the beginning of another turning point. By then I was feeling strong and safe enough to be able to confront and challenge those difficult feelings that experiences, such as the above, left me with. In some ways they were reminders of my adolescent experience of not fitting in and of feeling that those around me perceived my Arabic background as being inferior and uncivilized. With my defences becoming less rigid and my mind opening up again, I began to understand how deeply embedded, unconscious and institutionalized these beliefs and attitudes are, towards those who are different.

Like the consultant who, as a lead clinician for a child and family service serving a large ethnic minority community, told me 'you cannot work with these Asian families, the best you can hope is to save a few of their youngsters if you can get access to them'. Like the consultant who, perhaps oblivious to my background, commented in relation to Arabic countries 'I would hate to come from that background because of the way they treat their women'. Like the recurrent stereotypes family therapists at a well-known institution would remark thus on Asian families they were working with 'I think this father is domineering, controlling and oppressive/abusive both to his wife and his children'. Like the consultant who told an Arabic colleague of mine who had come to train as a child psychiatrist in the UK 'I cannot support your application for a senior registrar post or give you a reference as I believe our training schemes should be for UK graduates, not those from overseas'. Like the planning committee I sat on as an observer that was planning a study day on the mental-health problems of refugees; the committee was made up of eight people in management roles, all white, none of them with any personal experience of being a refugee, all the invited speakers were white, none of whom had any personal experience of being a refugee and no refugee organizations were consulted. Like the professor who commented when challenged about the lack of ethnic minority staff in her particular clinic, 'ethnic minority families often prefer to see white mental-health members of staff and do not wish to meet with a member from their own community, anyway there are too many languages spoken in this area so we will always end up discriminating against somebody'. Like an organization I worked with that employed several bilingual co-workers to act as health advocates, to learn from us and teach us about their communities, who nearly 2 years after first starting were being used rarely by other members of staff, and when they were used were used as interpreters only, leaving them feeling unvalued, marginalized and isolated. Like the number of management committees I have known operating in high ethnic-minority areas with no ethnic-minority membership or indeed consultation.

I could go on, this is just the tip of the iceberg and only deals with the issue of my personal experiences in relation to how institutionalized discriminatory beliefs are in many mental-health organizations. There is so much more that I have not touched on, like the detachment of the academic world, particularly in child and adolescent psychiatry, from the clinical one. Unscrupulous researchers in ivory towers turning everything into research projects for the sake of having their names in lights, producing research which is of dubious quality, has little user involvement and is of virtually no consequence or interest for those of us working in clinical settings. Like the power conversations that consultants have behind closed doors, where the arrogance really begins to show with the conviction that they are the most highly paid because they are the most intelligent, with the accompanying belief that this powerful status must be preserved at all costs.

Fortunately, during this time I have also met many therapists (including psychiatrists) who have been immensely influential in helping me open my horizons and develop my thinking. Like the consultant who told me 'patients hate therapists who cannot be themselves'. Like the black family therapist who had burned all her training books and papers, feeling that her training had said nothing to her about her background, culture and beliefs. She did not adhere to any western-style therapy structures or methods, yet she seemed to be popular and effective with her clients. Like the therapist who had a wonderful ability for noticing the positives and introduced me to narrative therapies and post-modern thinking. Like the consultant who herself was from an ethnic minority and a trained psychoanalyst, who helped me re-examine some of my psychoanalytic assumptions and under-stand the importance of ordinary people's everyday experiences. Indeed without all these positive, helpful influences, it would have been impossible to challenge and change my assumptions and thinking, and survive with some identity intact whilst working within western mental-health institutions.

Chapter 2

The post-modern landscape and children's mental health

Oh, my body, make of me always a man who questions.

(Frantz Fanon, 1967: 232)

Frantz Fanon (1967) spoke of a devastating pathology at the heart of western culture, that of a denial of difference. Of course many cultures struggle with difference, the alien, the outsider. But for the global colonizer, imposing their world view with all its assumptions and definitions of desirability, the consequent intimidation, belittling and pervading sense of inferiority for those who don't fit the powerful colonizer's definitions is something the colonizer need have little awareness of. The colonized either passively accepts their inferiority or bubbles into a seething cauldron of anger and madness.

In the modernist's view the world is made up of demonstrable and discoverable laws which can be applied to all aspects of life. In this view of things differences are not as important as 'discovering' similarities and creating universal laws to shape our understanding of the world and our place in it. Full of the hope and optimism born out of the real fruit of modernist medicine, doctors set out to conquer, understand and liberate the mind. In this universalistic, positivist, rationalist, scientific mode of enquiry they generated theory after theory, produced research paper after research paper and still the goods were not delivered. But cultural dominance was on their side. Common sense would have dictated a gradual demise of both the dominance and universalistic assumptions underlying the psychiatric approach to mental health. As Thomas Szasz (1987: 57) once stated

If psychiatrists had to pay interest on their promise of pathological lesions (to prove mental illness as a putative brain disease) as borrowers must to lenders, the interest alone would already have bankrupted them; instead they keep reissuing the same notes undaunted by their perfect record of never meeting their obligations.

(1987: 57)

But if you own the rights to define common sense then common sense will be twisted to your purpose. The modernists then stamped their authority further and so the development of children came to be scrutinized within a modernist, professional, universalistic, normal/pathological framework and the process of medicalizing, psychiatrizing and pathologizing differences amongst children got under way.

Then the world became more global. The colonized broke off their political shackles only to find the colonizer wise to this manœuvre and having already done enough to ensure that economic and cultural shackles remained. Mass movement of refugees occurred, societies were forced to face up to their multicultural nature and the media exploded images and messages daily into people's homes. The modernist project was no longer as easy, but they worked hard to keep the weight of cultural history, embedded as it is in the establishments that control, and thus further dominance was assured. Other voices, other views, differences in how we understand our world, life, its problems, growing up, normal, abnormal, had to shout loud to be heard. Child and adolescent psychiatry controls from within the comfort of its historical and material status tied as it is to the status of medicine. But those of us who can see through its superficiality must continue to raise our voices, challenge and question. Without this, the rearranging of deck chairs masquerading as progress will continue. Without this, the inherent racism and cultural colonialism will continue.

My wish is not to make a wholesale attack on child and adolescent psychiatry as a discipline that should be dumped. My wish is to question the assumptions, the universals, the constructs, the clinical applications and all those things that make up my job as a child and adolescent psychiatrist. I believe that as a profession we must be able to appreciate the relative nature of the belief systems we use in our work (and therefore hopefully be able to make positive use of other belief systems). We also must reflect on how our position as a very dominant and powerful agent in our society can have a profound effect, not only on the clients we work with, but on our modern cultural discourse about children, adolescents and families more generally.

In this chapter I hope to provide some theoretical context for the rest of the book. First I compare the modernist approaches that currently dominate theory, research and practice in child and adolescent psychiatry with what I believe to be a more realistic, flexible and open minded philosophical position, which incorporates post-modern thinking in particular. Much of the book involves deconstructing the dominant position that child and adolescent psychiatry holds. This involves turning the microscope away from its main object of study, the clients, and back on to our profession in order to analyse and understand child and adolescent psychiatry itself as a particular cultural grouping. Thus, the latter part of this chapter begins the process of understanding the influence of culture on my profession's territory, illustrating, hopefully, how important it is to recognize differences and how current theory and practice in child and adolescent psychiatry has failed to do this.

Modernist and post-modernist views

Roger Lowe (1991: 43) offers a succinct definition of post-modernism: 'in general terms post-modernism represents a radical questioning of the foundationalism and absolutism of modern conceptions of knowledge'. In the field of mental health this can be interpreted as the idea that no one person or approach has the definitive answer.

Let me briefly compare this approach to the modernist approach that dominates current theory and practice in child and adolescent mental health and indeed the mental-health movement more generally. Modernism holds that we are capable of arriving at a universally true, objective reality that separates objective fact from the subjective world. Modernism privileges a steadily growing body of what it believes to be objective knowledge (Freedman and Combs, 1996). This idea that there are common, fundamental, universal, psychological characteristics common to all humans is traceable in modern, western thought to the early enlightenment era (Jahoda, 1990). The influence and successes of scientific biology, the Darwinian evolutionary perspective and medical science has no doubt had a big influence on the development of similar universalistic law discovering approaches to the knowledge base in mental health.

The modernist approach to mental health essentially entails the observation of persons in order to compare their thoughts, feelings and behaviours against a pre-existing assumed normal. The modernist practitioner then plans her/his interventions to try and change the person(s) in a way that brings their thoughts, feelings and behaviours closer to this assumed normal. This approach to the field of subjective human experience brings with it some fundamental problems. First, the modernist practitioners define themselves apart from their clients. They can sustain the belief that they are the experts with special knowledge that allows them to observe, assess, diagnose and treat without the practitioner having reason to believe that they themselves are subject to and part of the same human processes as the person with whom they are interacting. For the modernist, the observer is distinct from the person(s) being observed (Keeney, 1983). Furthermore, the locus for understanding a person's complex life is assumed to be lodged with the practitioner (the expert) not the client. Second, the modernist practitioner, by ignoring the ever present dimensions of power in social life, is not only inadvertently sustaining potentially oppressive relations of power (Goldner, 1985; Hare-Mustin, 1978; Pare, 1996) but also discarding and ignoring rich and useful other sources for understanding and generating solutions to a problem. Third, the modernist practitioner by virtue of her/his status, privileges their own professional knowledge and thereby contributes to the process of professionalization of common human experiences and to building a cultural discourse that can undermine peoples' own capacity to make sense of their lives and find solutions to their problems. Fourth, by promoting the idea that scientific certainty exists in the field of subjective human experience, modernist practitioners contribute to a discourse that stifles diversity, devalues difference and in its most extreme form represents a kind of eugenic terrorism.

Despite the hype, a modernist approach to knowledge in the field of mental health has been unable to claim the successes seen in other spheres of life. Post-modern thinking questions whether the modern ordering of phenomena which claims to be autonomous to the situation of the knower, deserves to be privileged over an ordering of phenomena that is orientated by the situation of the knower. We must begin to appreciate that the knowledge of the knower is not a disinterested mental representation of external reality, of some absolute truth (Inden, 1990). The limits of usefulness of universalistic, positivist knowledge reverberate through into many of the allied disciplines and theory bases that we use in mental health. Byrne and Kelley (1992) conclude that socio-biological research on human psychology is based on loosely assembled principles that can be stretched and bent to accommodate most empirical findings. There is often a tendency to assume that the mere existence of a particular behaviour means that it has some adaptive value with consequent leaps of faith that confuse observed behaviour with genetic biological imperatives (Bombar, 1996). Furthermore, psychological, social and psychiatric literature is full of the universalistic tendency of interpreting any similarities across culture as implying biological causation, ignoring possible shared psychological, ecological, social and cultural structures (Kagitcibasi, 1996). This also dismisses the different potential meanings we can ascribe to similar behaviours that can have a huge impact on the way we approach our professional practice.

Arguably, most of the world have been and continue to be skeptical about cold positivist, metaphors for understanding the world around us. In Europe and North America, so called post-modern thinking (I use this term loosely and interchangeably with what has also been called social constructionist or post-structuralist approaches) has challenged traditional western, modernist assumptions. Post-modern thinking highlighted those traditional versions of materialism, determinism and realism, which have generated confident universalistic knowledge claims about the world and are always problematic. It has argued that knowledge is a set of representations and, particularly when applied to what might loosely be termed subjective reality, it is a map and not the territory itself, in other words modernism often confuses the idea with the thing itself. In relation to the mental-health industry, post-modern thinkers have been particularly critical to the point of suggesting that in some instances modernist approaches to mental health cannot be regarded as a source of progress but as a basis for alienation (Foucault, 1965; Cushman, 1995; Anderson, 1990; Berger and Luckman, 1967; Neimeyer and Mahoney, 1995; Sarbin and Kitsuse, 1994; Shotter, 1993; Parry and Doon, 1994; Parker et al., 1995). More broadly post-modern thinkers have suggested that it is no longer possible to generate universal solutions and answers to the problems and questions of contemporary forms of life. They argue that the analysis, understanding, goals and values which have been central to western European civilization since enlightenment can no longer be assumed to be universally valid or indeed relevant (Lyotard, 1986; Harvey, 1989; Arac, 1989). Thus, from the starting point that when people live in the world differently it may be that they live in different worlds

(Shweder, 1991), various mental-health professionals have used post-modern thinking as a legitimate set of ideas which can be used to begin analysing current theory and practice. Under such analysis the focus begins to turn from exclusively examining apparent exterior objectivity to looking at the interior subjectivity of the meaning giver.

One particular problem with this approach is that it can give the impression that all explanations are simply of equal value. This is clearly not the case. It is important to take into account the fact that different systems may prove to be of different worth. For example, in most of physical medicine there is a greater capacity to arrive at objective facts using a modernist knowledge base than there is in psychiatry and psychology. Thus, a more critical approach to post-modern thinking will inevitably result in biased value judgements as some sources of knowledge are inevitably more privileged over others. This has led some to talk about working with preferred meanings (Giroux, 1983; Waldegrave, 1990; Hindmarsh, 1993; Tamasese and Waldegrave, 1993), in other words meanings that emerge out of values. For example, perpetrators and survivors of childhood sexual abuse may well give very different meanings to the events of an episode of abuse, but this does not mean that these meanings should be given equal value. We are likely to take a value judgement as to which of the two meanings we wish to privilege and whose voice we wish to amplify (Bograd, 1984; Goldner, 1985; McKinnon *et al.*, 1987; Kamsler, 1990).

The post-modern practitioner is no longer the expert knowing how people should behave, think, feel and solve their difficulties. Instead, she/he is committed to a side-by-side, less hierarchical, therapeutic relationship, with the practitioner finding ways to honour and privilege the client's own abilities to locate fresh directions and solutions to their problems. They focus less on what they assume to be abnormal or pathological and more on alternatives to the problem-saturated story (White and Epston, 1990) through careful listening and responding to the client's own knowledge (Weingarten, 1998).

It is important to keep the idea of post-modern thinking itself in some sort of context. When post-modern critique attacks the universality and validity of concepts used in mental health (for example diagnosis) this does not mean that the behaviour being classified or the distress that may be accompanying these behaviours is not being recognized. The situation is not that these problems do not exist but how they should be meaningfully interpreted, for it is the interpretation and meaning one assigns an experience or behaviour that involves making all sorts of assumptions which are very often culturally specific (Laungani, 1992). Furthermore, we should remember that the struggle to understand the world directly does produce worthwhile and helpful maps. What I believe we must continue to do however, is to be questioning, critical and skeptical towards those attitudes and assumptions so prevalent in modernist mental-health literature that these maps are the territory and are necessarily the most superior source of knowledge (Bhaskar, 1989; Greenwood, 1994; Pilgrim and Rogers, 1994).

Interpreting meaning

To begin to grapple with and conceptualize different systems of knowledge for understanding and dealing with child and adolescent mental-health problems it is helpful to gain some understanding of how different cultural systems of knowledge focus on, value and privilege different things. One useful starting point is to reflect on general differences between cultures by conceptualizing them as continuums within various dimensions.

Several authors have written about different dimensional models to help conceptualize cross-cultural values and perceptions. For example, Hofstede (1980, 1983, 1994a, 1994b) developed five largely independent dimensions to help interpret results of cross-cultural empirical studies in social science. The dimensions described were individualism–collectivism, power–distance, uncertainty–avoidance, masculinity–femininity and Confucian–dynamism. Although this scheme has been influential particularly in cross-cultural psychology studies there are many other different schemes for classifying cultural dimensions. For example, Douglas (1970a, 1982) whilst also embodying concepts of individualism–collectivism and hierarchy also classifies on a dimension of mastery–egalitarianism. Similarly, within the field of mental health, differences particularly between western and non-western cultures have also been analysed using a dimensional approach. For example Waldegrave (1997) conceptualizes differences between Maori/Pacific Island and European values along the dimensions of communal–individual, spiritual–secular, ecological–consumer and consensual–conflictual. Fernando (1995) conceptualizes differences between western cultures' reactions to problems to do with thinking, feelings, fears, anxieties and so on, and eastern approaches to these problems along the continuums of self-sufficiency versus integration and harmony, personal autonomy versus social integration, efficiency versus balanced functioning and self esteem versus protection. Many of these dimensional models are being used to illustrate that values and orientation to understanding meaning are sometimes in dialectical opposition between western and non-western cultures.

One of the most widely discussed dimensions that is common to nearly all the dimensional conceptualizations of cross-cultural difference is that of the individual orientation as opposed to the collectivist or family orientation within a culture. Individualism is very characteristic of western cultures and the ideologies it generates, including that of child and adolescent psychiatry. Individualized cultures are those where individuals are viewed as loosely connected, with each looking after their own interests or those of their immediate family (Hofstede, 1994a). Where there is a conflict between these interests and those of their social or kinship grouping, individuals put their personal goals first (Singelis *et al.*, 1995). Individualist orientations emphasize personal autonomy and the 'I' (Yang, 1981; Triandis, 1995). Individuals in such cultures find it easier to detach themselves from family, community and religion. They may change friends and marital partners more freely with rational principles and norms forming the basis of their interactions (Kim, 1994; Triandis, 1995).

In contrast, in collectivist societies people from birth onwards are integrated into strong, cohesive groups which continue to protect them in exchange for loyalty throughout a person's life (Hofstede, 1994b). The 'we' dominates with obligations and duties often overriding personal preferences in importance (Triandis, 1995). In such a system marriage links families, not just individuals, and a person is seen as part of the embedded, interconnectedness of relationships (Shweder and Bourne, 1982; Strathern, 1992). I will return to this issue later in this chapter when I look more closely at how these, sometimes opposing, sets of cultural values, beliefs and practices influence our beliefs with regard to child rearing, as well as our understanding of what constitutes a problem in children's development and how this should be dealt with.

Of course, it is important not to reduce these differences to stereotypes, as within all cultures there is great variety of values and experiences once a person experiences a particular culture close up. Any person's culture is also interacting with his or her own individual personality and world views (Rogoff and Chavajay, 1995). Within any nation there are also important cultural groupings, for example between different social classes, where an enormous variety of psychological functioning and belief systems can be found (Kohn *et al.*, 1990). Neither is any culture a stationary static thing, but a constantly changing dynamic. Cultures across the world are constantly undergoing political and demographic transition (for example, so called globalization). These macro system changes also impact on people's behaviour and their models of thought about their behaviour. Thus, when trying to understand cultural models it is also important to take into account the fact that people's views are interdependent with their micro and macro environment (Trickett and Buchanan, 1997; Bronfenbrenner, 1970; Berry, 1994).

Using such a cross-cultural and anthropological perspective to look at and analyse my own profession it is possible and, I believe, valid to conceptualize child and adolescent psychiatry as a cultural group with its own history of ideas, beliefs and values which powerfully contributes to the clinicians' theory and practice. Western mental-health culture is naturally dominated by concepts derived from western, modernist approaches to understanding life and its problems. This means that in most western countries (and, unfortunately, in many developing countries too), people from indigenous and ethnic minorities who wish to enter the mental-health professions are expected to gain a western-conceived and dominated qualification. To do this often requires that they leave their communities, values and traditions to study a system of thinking that uses thinking and theories based on different, often culturally colonial, values and beliefs in order to be qualified to work with their own culture again. This is a model for a form of cultural colonialism that I believe child and adolescent mental-health training and services are guilty of perpetuating.

Discourse and power

Our professional training, just as with other cultural activities, provides us with stories or scripts which we use to make sense of and interpret the meaning of the problems our clients come with. It also shapes the development of the interventions that we use in our daily professional lives.

Our professional cultural lives are surrounded by these discourses which are made up not only of content and silences of texts, conversations and other sources of information, but of tried practices too. The fabric of our social world of discourse often determines what behaviours are considered acceptable and unacceptable as well as which ideas and people are deemed relevant and worth following and which ones are thought of as being on the fringe. This fabric is shaped by those with the power to determine such things and is not easily unravelled (Monk *et al.*, 1997). Clearly, some people have more power to make meaning than others do. It is important to understand that certain versions of knowledge that emerge in any local discourse are likely to reflect the power differentials between different groups in any given local context. Knowledge and reality are not only socially constructed but are also the dominant systems of knowledge used, and reflect the dominance of one or more particular groups over others.

The way power hierarchies have influenced and dominated local knowledge can be readily understood by examining the process of colonization. In his study of the colonization of Egypt, Mitchell (1988) traced how colonization involved gradually changing many precolonial epistemologies through the scientific cataloguing of reality and by constructing versions of personhood through an opposition between interior and exterior. This was a process that continually undermined and belittled the local values, ways of organizing life and constructions of personhood (Mitchell, 1988). The colonizer uses various myths, fantasies and ideologies to maintain a division between the colonizer and the colonized (Delal, 1993). Ethnic minority cultures have therefore often been described in a way that makes them seem backward or bizarre, or in a way that implied that their problems are somehow caused by the very nature of their culture (Mares *et al.*, 1985).

To this day, the very fabric of our society is permeated by such an attitude which can manifest itself in education, media, history books, social work, psychotherapies, children's stories and psychiatric practice, to name but a few. Therapies, psychiatric, psychological and social practices are soaked in this kind of cultural imperialism which, I believe, is a kind of cultural racism whereby the cultures of groups other than the white, western, middle-class definers of normality are seen in inferior, deficient and pathological terms. For many clients, and indeed professionals, who refuse to turn their back on their own cultural beliefs and practices (which are being viewed as inferior and pathological), any lack of therapeutic success or any experience of discrimination is often then interpreted as their own fault (Massey, 1991). These days colonization is not carried out through the barrel of a gun as often as it is carried out through the words and discourses that dominate and control the hearts, minds and spirits of people all over the world. My profession is certainly not immune to this process. On the contrary, like other institutions born out of dominant western philosophy and beliefs, it is soaked in it and sometimes drunk with the power this gives it.

Culture and child rearing

The closer anyone gets to lived experience of real people the more variety is encountered both between cultures and within any culture. Having made this important point I would like to briefly explore some generalized differences in child-rearing approaches, beliefs and values that are often encountered when a cross-cultural perspective is taken. For the sake of brevity and because of limitations of space, I will start by focusing on a frequently discussed aspect, which is the difference between individualist (mainly western) orientated cultures and collectivist orientated cultures.

The western, individualist approach to child rearing places value on fostering independence, autonomy, self-determination, separation, individuation and self-expression. Parents are often at pains to make their children independent as quickly as possible with an emphasis on fostering this as early in life as possible (Roland, 1980). Although the process of colonizing the world meant making others dependent, being dependent has come to be viewed as a shameful state of being and a cause for grave social concern. This is reflected in the professional literature on child development, with analysis of children's psychological and psychiatric problems and how to deal with them centreing around how to foster independence in the client's children, often seeing this as the most important aspect of their work (Dwivedi, 1995b). Children are expected to have their own voices, preferably with clear differences being apparent from that of their parents (Dwivedi, 1995b). At a family level in modern individualist cultures the family is viewed as independent of its kin, content to go it alone, often with roles and positions in the family becoming unclear (Kagitcibasi, 1996). Some have commented that this increasing psychological separation between children and their families has also led to increasing inconsistencies in child rearing with the disappearance of clear-cut role models (e.g. Sinha, 1988) and the consequent greater professionalization of the whole area of child rearing. However, it has also been noted that many families, particularly those making the transition from more collectivist cultures to western ones, often adapt to changing circumstances and find a way to allow old traditional values to fit in with the new valued aspirations found in the host community (Bradley and Weisner, 1997; Vergin, 1985; Cha, 1994).

In contrast, collectivist cultures place more emphasis on the notion of dependability. Parents are often at pains to ensure their children grow up with adults who are models of dependability. For many collectivist societies kinship is the single most important cultural institution, organizing careers, marriages and even personal identities. In the west the concept of kinship is based primarily on biological relationships, whereas in many other societies the concept is broader and incorporates the wider religious and social community (Sow, 1985). For example, in some native American Indian tribes a person may refer to some twenty people as their mother and consider one hundred or more people as brothers and sisters (Stanton, 1995). Many collectivist societies encourage obedience to authority and interdependence with others (Ellis and Petersen, 1992). Family obligations are often highly ritualized with a relative lack of importance given to an individual's own opinions (Hoffstede, 1994b).

To help flesh this picture out, I will give a brief outline of some child-rearing characteristics in a few predominantly collectivist cultures.

In many Arab and Middle Eastern societies traditional child-rearing practices foster behaviour orientated towards interdependence rather than individuation and independence. Children are encouraged to express their emotions as opposed to developing self-control over them. By western standards the behaviour of parents towards their children would seem enmeshed and intrusive. Mothers, for example, tend to have a great readiness to interest themselves in their children's affairs. Traditional Arab beliefs view the bond between mother and child as unseverable. The father's role may be seen as more distant but is no less important. As head of the family he insists on good behaviour, and fears being blamed should one of his children become delinquent or premaritally pregnant. Indeed it is one of the duties of Islam to provide good discipline for the children (Timimi, 1995). Within a household the children's mother is often viewed as a broker or mediator between the children and their father, the mother meanwhile often influences other members of the family through the agency of her eldest son (Bouhdiba, 1977). The clear-cut roles with a hierarchy built around age and gender, operating with the expectation that as children go through adolescence conflicts between individual needs and aspirations and family needs are resolved predominantly in the interests of family loyalty, has led to Arab culture being described as characterized by hierarchy and ambivalence as opposed to autonomy and conflict which characterize western nuclear families (Davis and Davis, 1989). Ambivalence is frequently encountered in adolescence and young adulthood where mood changes associated with puberty are widely recognized and tolerated. However, the maturing individual is expected to reorganize unmet personal aspirations so as not to conflict with parental expectation. In return the parents are expected to actively help their offspring with life tasks such as finding work and a suitable marriage partner. Thus, psychological theories describing adolescence as a stage of involving autonomy and independence bear only limited relevance to the common patterns of psychosocial maturation encountered in Arabic culture (Gilligan, 1982; Ammar, 1973).

Traditional Indian culture bears many similarities to Arab culture, particularly in its emphasis on the closeness of a child to its mother, which has been idealized throughout Indian, particularly Hindu, culture. Early child rearing has been described as conducted in an atmosphere of indulgence, physical closeness, common sleeping arrangements and immediate gratification of physical and emotional needs. This often leads to a prolonged babyhood compared with western culture, with an overriding attitude that young children are to be loved just for being, rather than for doing the right things (Kumar, 1992). This luxurious indulgence, however, doesn't last for ever, often being disrupted by the birth of a new sibling or by what has been described as the phenomena of 'the second birth'. This occurs at about 4 or 5 years old when the expectations placed upon children radically change (Carstairs, 1957). At these ages gender roles may become more starkly demarcated, with girls being given more household chores and boys being expected to show more socially responsive behaviour. The extended family system often means that there is a certain amount of psychosocial diffusion. Thus, a father is often found to be restrained in the presence of his own son(s), in the interests of being able to divide his attention and support equally between his own and his brother's sons (Kakar, 1978). Similarly, many mothers will refer not only to their own biological offspring but also to offspring of sisters-in-law, sisters and even friends as their children (Trawick, 1990). A marked preference for sons over daughters in traditional Indian families is common. Sons are necessary to complete some Hindu religious rituals and are also economically more valuable as they will bring brides (often with financially valuable dowries) into the family. At the same time there is abundant allusion to the warmth, intimacy and relaxed affection that exists, particularly between a mother and her daughter in Indian culture (Ross, 1961). Some of the resentment that exists amongst women about the clear preference of sons over daughters is reflected in some aspects of female culture in Indian society, such as in popular songs and jokes where women do react against the discrimination of their culture, portraying men as vain, faithless and infantile (Gupta, 1970). At the same time it has been noted that many Indian women seem to be conservative defenders of the current system of family life (Kakar, 1978). The reason for this may relate to the identity conferred to women once they become mothers. Motherhood appears (for some) to hold the solution to many of the previous difficulties a woman may have encountered. Tasks are removed, affection and care may visibly increase and a new mother's social standing changes (Kakar, 1978).

In Chinese societies the family is also the central, basic unit of society (Xantian, 1985) and is central to self-identity (Hsu, 1985). Many of the basic beliefs and values concerning family life has been heavily influenced by the teaching of Confucius which dates back to the fifth century BC (Meredith and Abbott, 1995). Confucius teaches individuals to value the collective welfare of the family more than the individual and to take responsibility in community affairs (Schneider et al., 1997). Traditional extended family systems are believed to provide not only material security but also the psychological security of ancestral lineage (Chu, 1985). This philosophy has led to the development of various practical and educational developments in child-rearing patterns in such societies. For example, it is common for young children to continue sleeping with their mother or sometimes grandmother for many years (Lau, 1996). Childhood stories, often with religious underpinnings, are also regularly told to children from a young age and stress the importance of family and family interdependence (Lau, 1996). These attitudes continue to influence such that self-realization is not seen as being as important as developing broader social responsibility, as the child enters into adulthood (King and Bond, 1985). A son's respect for his father may involve continued displays of obedience throughout that son's life (Hsu, 1983; Wolf, 1996). For example, he may be obliged to make continued financial contributions to the parents even after leaving home (Argyle, 1982). In return parental nurture and support continues well after the child has grown up (Yang, 1988).

Not only do different societies around the world develop different general sets of values and beliefs that influence their attitudes and practices concerning family life and child rearing, but it is also possible to identify many important and significant differences within cultures too. For example, Kohn (1987 et al., 1990) has argued that the social-class position of parents greatly affects the opportunities for occupational self-direction and control. Thus, middle-class parents are more likely than working-class parents to value self-direction in their children and espouse beliefs in child rearing consistent with these values (Tudge et al., 1997). In some countries, particularly in rural, non-industrialized areas, children's material help is considered particularly important in family life (Kagitcibasi, 1982). In such situations it could be argued that childhood as a distinct entity becomes less evident (Kagitcibasi, 1996).

These cultural differences are of more than just passing academic interest to the clinician as they highlight the importance of understanding the belief framework of the interpreter of behaviour to appreciate what meaning and significance certain childhood behaviours are afforded. In many instances it can be seen that the same behaviours by the child may be differently interpreted in different cultures (Orlick et al., 1990). The child who dresses him or herself may be seen by an Israeli mother as demonstrating independence but by a Japanese mother as demonstrating obedience (Heath, 1995). Parental control may be perceived as hostility and rejection in North America, whilst in Japan and Korea may be seen as warmth and acceptance (Kagitcibasi, 1996). These differences are so fundamental that it has become apparent that the problem of interpreting the meaning and significance of children's behaviours makes even the idea of defining the basic rights of children an interpretive minefield. The UN convention on the rights of the child (United Nations General Assembly, 1989) has sought to codify children's protection and rights. Yet cultural differences in how to interpret these rights have been evident from the start and reflect the different emphasis given in child-rearing beliefs and practices in different cultures (Murphy-Berman et al., 1996). Saks (1996), in a study of differences in the interpretation of the convention, gave delegates from eleven different countries attending a convention meeting a list of ten different child-rearing practices (including such things as corporal punishment and the right of parents to insist that a 14-year-old follows the parents' religious belief). Saks then asked the delegates whether the convention permitted these ten different practices or not. On all but one of the ten items there was disagreement about whether the convention allowed this practice or not.

Culture and pathology

Just as important differences in child rearing exist between cultures so important differences also exist in the way different cultural groups understand and interpret problems. In many non-western cultures the mind/body dichotomy does not dominate thinking about human life and its problems. In many other cultures, matters brought together in psychiatry in the west are seen in religious, spiritual, social, political, philosophical, psychological, ethical or medical terms (or indeed various mixtures of these) (Fernando, 1995). In particular the importance of the spiritual realm to the types of problems commonly categorized as psychiatric can be seen in many non-western cultures. For example, in many African societies it is taught that reality consists in the relation not of men (and women) with things but of men (and women) with other men (and women) and of all men (and women) with the spiritual world (Lambo, 1969).

The lack of differentiation between mind and body is reflected in the basic philosophical underpinnings of many ancient, traditional forms of medicine. For example in Ayurvedic medicine (which has been traced as far back as 600 BC), psychic and somatic complaints and components of health, which are isolated from one another in western medicine, are integrated (Langford, 1995). Ayurvedic medicine conceives the body and person as fluid, penetrable and engaged with continuous interchange with the social and natural environment (Zimmerman, 1987; Kakar, 1982). While biomedicine sees illness as a discrete entity, Ayurvedic philosophy sees illness as a disruption in the delicate somatic, climactic and social systems of balance (Kakar, 1982; Trawick, 1991). Causes are not located as such but seen as part of a system out of balance. Symptoms are viewed as being part of a process rather than a disease entity (Obeyesekere, 1977).

Another ancient system of health and medicine is the Unani system practised in many Arab countries as well as in Indo-Pakistan. The basic philosophy of Unani (or Tibb) medicine is that the body is taken as a whole because harmonious life is possible only when there is a proper balance between physical and spiritual functions. In the Unani system of treatment great reliance is placed on the power of self-preservation and adjustment with the aim of the physician often being that of helping to develop these natural functions (Said, 1983).

Not only do different cultures and societies develop different systems for understanding and dealing with what we, in the west, would call psychological or psychiatric problems, but in addition many authors have suggested that different cultures' values and belief systems (particularly different cultures approach to self) can also be a factor in causing certain mental-health problems. For example, eating disorders are most commonly identified in societies with a strong ideal of self-cherishing and fear of fatness. When eating disorders do occur in women from societies who do not cherish these values they are often described as being associated with self-renunciation rather than the western ideal of a desire for slimness (Littlewood, 1995). Some have argued that every age develops its own particular forms of pathology, which express in exaggerated form that era's underlying character structure. Thus, in Freud's time hysteria and obsessional neurosis carried to extremes the personality traits associated with the capitalist order at an earlier stage in its development with its fanatical devotion to work and fierce repression of sexuality (Dwivedi, 1996). In our time the preschizophrenic, borderline and narcissistic personality disorders have attracted increasing attention, along with schizophrenia itself (Lasch, 1980). The rising tide of so-called narcissistic disorders in western culture may be, in part, because many western societies regard narcissism as a goal not a problem. Manipulation of personal relationships, the discouragement of deep personal attachments and the enhancement of self-fulfillment are traits that can be adaptive to the modern management culture (Solomon, 1990).

Culture and treatment

If we hold on to universalistic assumptions concerning child rearing and pathology, not only are we in danger of imposing inappropriate frameworks that may, in some instances, lead to a worsening of problems, but we are also depriving ourselves as clinicians from the opportunities, possibilities and creativity that can arise from being able to take and use alternative viewpoints and frameworks.

At the superficial level it can be seen that professionals who follow theories centred around the importance of fostering autonomy and independence can soon alienate clients from cultures where autonomy is less valued (Buunk and Hupka, 1986). In addition any interventions must also be seen against the backdrop of economic and social reality. For example, child psychiatry in India is likely to be very different in its priorities and needs to those found in the west, as the problems of poverty are more basic and fundamental to the problems of living than in the west (Ujjwalarani, 1992). It also needs to be recognized that interventions in this field of personal human relationships inevitably involve value judgements. To be effective means to be ready to find out what people want and to 'get your hands dirty' by trying to engage, understand and act upon relevant cultural, social and moral issues (Kagitcibasi, 1991). As clinicians we have to, in order to take on the perspective of different belief systems, suspend some of our own culturally conditioned and deeply held beliefs. Such a letting go is, of course, extremely difficult (Dwivedi, 1997). We know that many professionals in child and adolescent mental health have a primary aim of fostering independent views and opinions so that children appear to have their own voices (Dwivedi, 1995a). Sometimes, if a child or adolescent does not express such independent views, it can raise concern and may lead to professionals intervening and interpreting that the youngster's family has been repressive. The more we impose such value judgements as if they were already some universal truth, the more we risk many ethnic minority children's (and children from other social groups such as children from working-class families) difficulties being further exacerbated by professionals who unwittingly conflate culturally different value systems with psychopathology. Sometimes the damage to self-identity in such a climate, given that it replicates the colonizer/colonized dynamic (and similar power dynamics that often accompany this such as superior/inferior, clever/ stupid, healthy/unhealthy and so on), is extremely difficult to repair (Dwivedi, 1993a, 1993b, 1995b).

Different belief systems and values repeatedly challenge our own professional ethics and frameworks. Some families from other cultures may only feel comfortable in talking about intimate matters if they can approach the therapist as kin or, at the very least, as a friend, thereby challenging common professional ideas about boundaries (Bang, 1987; Miatra and Miller, 1996). If you cannot adapt to this you risk not only alienating the family but worse, pathologizing them for such attitudes and creating a climate where therapeutic progress becomes impossible. To further broaden and enrich our professional western, mental-health ideologies in child and adolescent psychiatry, we need to seek to embrace, explore and give at least equal value to different cultures' own indigenous theories (Gergen *et al.*, 1996; Heelas and Lock, 1981).

Professional culture

Thus we come full circle in this chapter. Having examined how other systems of thought conceptualize and understand children and their problems with reference to the power dynamic that privileges certain scripts, we return to the question of the inadequacy of modernist, professional psychiatric culture in addressing and understanding the problems of child and adolescent mental health. For progressive development to occur professional culture has to move beyond the current, narrow, medical model and other western therapy model-derived frameworks. Many have already criticized the lack of acknowledgement within psychiatry of the relative nature of its theories. Some have gone further, for example Szasz (1961, 1987) asserted that psychiatry has produced no genuine problem-solving accomplishment. He regarded psychiatry as a pseudo-science, a rhetorical enterprise masquerading as a medical or scientific one. He saw psychiatry as having a hidden social and political agenda, which, through the rhetoric of diagnosis and treatment of mental illness and disorders, functioned to accredit socially valued behaviour and discredit socially unvalued behaviour. He noted that the medical model has not transformed psychiatry and that we seem no closer to finding the real, presumed biological causes of any of the major mental illnesses that psychiatry diagnoses.

Fernando (1988) conceptualizes the culture of psychiatry as being built around certain core features that have arisen from western philosophy, namely the mind–body dichotomy, a mechanistic view of life, materialistic concept of mind, a segmented approach to the individual, biomedical change as illness and natural causes of illness. Unlike the rest of medicine though, psychiatry has arguably not delivered with these principles and this framework. For example, in relation to the biggest preoccupation of biological psychiatrists, Barnes (1987: 433) concludes 'for every point about the biology of schizophrenia there is a counter point. Theories about the origin and disease process of schizophrenia are often built on a multitude of empirical observations and a paucity of hard facts.' Similarly, on this same question, Lieberman and Koreen (1993: 425) conclude 'a fragmentary body of data which provides neither consistent nor conclusive evidence for any specific aetiological theory'. Despite this lack of evidence and despite the conclusion of many well meaning 'eclectic' practitioners that schizophrenia is thus more likely to be multifactorial in origin, there is still the basic assumption that a biological substratum underlies the change within the individual and that schizophrenia is best conceptualized as 'mental illness' (Fernando, 1995).

Child and adolescent psychiatry originates from a similar set of philosophical value judgements and needs to be critically evaluated in a similar manner. As seen through a post-modern lens, child and adolescent psychiatrists and other mental-health professionals dealing with childhood are immersed in predominant cultural influences and ideologies with knowledge and solutions for mental-health problems as biased and subjective as those of their clients. Shotter (1993) suggests that psychology (and the mental-health field generally) should be viewed as a 'moral' rather than 'natural' science – to reflect its interpretive underpinning and lack of universally valid objective knowledge. Similarly, Cushman (1995) criticizes traditional approaches to therapy for assuming an insulated, scientific, philosophy-free and value-free perch. Professionals who remain consistently unaware of the relative nature of their views, and naïvely assume that there is one reality and one right view, often incorrectly assume anyone who sees things differently must be either mad or bad (Watzlawick, 1976). Professionals in child and adolescent mental health use their diagnostic categories and subsequent interventions to honour only therapists' definitions of reality and health – clients are not usually welcome members in this club (Griffith and Griffith, 1994).

The power to define and own a kind of universal idea of normality and pathology has a massive effect, not only in its cultural ripples into everyday culture and language, but in the professionals' everyday work. The professional may be so convinced of the truth of their theoretical frame that it becomes unquestionable and unavailable for discussion. Thus, the professional may be more likely to attribute pathology or resistance to the client and not ever to the theoretical frame itself, if the client finds the professional's ideas unsuitable.

As Hoffman suggests

> For me, the most serious challenge to the field of mental health follows the post modern argument that much normal social science perpetuates a kind of colonial mentality in the minds of academics and practitioners. Therapists of all kinds must now investigate how relations of domination and submission are built into the very assumptions on which their practices are based.
>
> (1991: 9)

Chapter 3

Science and faith in mental health

When clients come to see a professional they hold a set of beliefs about the nature of their problem that is derived from those aspects of their culture with which they can identify. When professionals see clients the same process occurs, that is the professional develops a set of beliefs about the nature of the client's problem that is derived from those aspects of professional culture with which they can identify.

Cross-cultural observations

When I do presentations on cross-cultural approaches to child mental health I often start with a case history that goes something like this.

You are asked by a casualty doctor to carry out an urgent assessment on a 15-year-old boy (whom I shall refer to as 'A'). He has presented to casualty complaining of shortness of breath, dizziness, palpitations and a feeling that he was going to die. He had been investigated and nothing physically untoward was found. He then started crying, praying and clinging to a staff nurse pleading not to be sent home. Casualty staff expressed concern that he may be psychotic. When you assess him you find out the following. He is the youngest in a family of seven children. Both his parents come from Algeria. The family has been in the UK for 4 years. Prior to that they had spent 3 years in France, after leaving Algeria 7 years ago because of (according to them) political persecution. The boy dates his difficulties to about a year earlier when, according to him, his world fell apart. He describes the events leading up to this. He tells you that before this 'breakdown' he felt unsettled at his school, was changing peer group from time to time, sometimes being with a peer group that were getting into mild delinquency such as petty theft, drinking alcohol, smoking cannabis and engaging in gang fights. He describes becoming self-conscious about the colour of his skin at this time, feeling he is much darker than those around him are, even though he is living in quite a multicultural area. He describes becoming obsessed with a white girl in his class whom he wanted to date. Despite hearing from a friend that this girl would only go out with white boys he decided to ask her out on a date. The girl politely turned him down. He describes his life as turning upside down at this point. 'A' sees this as a major crossroads in his life. He felt his world began to fall apart. He couldn't eat or sleep.

At night he would lie awake crying. He began questioning many things about himself, his life, his attitudes, his family, his friends, his beliefs, his behaviour, and his ambitions. He withdrew from his circle of friends and stopped attending college. 'A' then decided he needed to turn to his religion, which he had neglected for many years, in the hope of finding answers. He started attending Islamic classes again and went back to the local mosque to reacquaint himself with an old peer group. He explains that during this period he came to realize he was on a very wayward path. 'A' then became very involved in religion asking for a sign from god (Allah) to guide him. After many weeks of looking, he realized his mistake. He realized that Allah does not respond to people who make demands. To gain the knowledge, he needed to submit to Allah's will. He describes how at this point of realization, an emotional floodgate opened and he felt Allah's presence like a bright light inside him. He then decided that his real calling was with Islam and that he should begin to dedicate himself to gaining more knowledge about Islam and to teaching others about his religion. Then an incident happened a few weeks ago. He was with some friends at the house of a school acquaintance, a young female teenager, talking about Islam. The father of this girl, on returning home, acted in a hostile manner towards him and his friends and they decided to flee the house running. 'A' then recalls seeing a number of what he believes are strange but significant events happening as they ran from this house. A black dog barking suddenly appeared and then disappeared. They ran past a tree with a strange artefact hanging from its branches. 'A' explained these to be signs that a djinn (a spirit) is active and waiting to prey on his vulnerable state. He tells you that he believes that at that moment a djinn entered into him. A couple of days later, as he was walking down the road, 'A' began to hear whisperings in his ear of a blasphemous nature. 'A' believed that these whisperings that he could hear were not coming from his own mind or thoughts but must be the result of the presence of the djinn in his body trying to posses him. He explains to you that since then he has experienced a number of things that have confirmed the djinn's presence, including pains in his abdomen, down his leg and in his genitalia, and dreams of an entity with claws digging deep into his body. He tells you that today he came to casualty after a distressing dream in which he believes there was evidence that the djinn was trying to kill him. He still believes that this djinn was trying to kill him.

You speak briefly to one of 'A's brothers who had come along with him. He tells you that they don't know why 'A' has been behaving so strangely recently. They are very concerned, as, for the past few weeks, he has not been sleeping at night, often coming into his parent's room in the middle of the night with tears in his eyes, unable to say why he is crying. His appetite has been poor and in his opinion 'A' has lost some weight. The brother confirms much of 'A's' history and tells you that he thinks 'A' hasn't been right for a good few months now. His brother believes that 'A' has got too deeply into religion and can't handle it. He tells you that 'A' has largely withdrawn from family life complaining about various family members' 'lack of religion'. He tells you that they are a very close family, having been brought closer by the difficult circumstances surrounding their migration from Algeria 7 years ago when their father was convinced that his life was in danger and that the Algerian secret service was after him. He tells you that since then their father has needed a lot of looking after and doesn't sleep well. He also tells you that a couple of years earlier their eldest sister, following a failed marriage, became possessed by a djinn. An imam from their local mosque was called and he helped them find a religious healer who successfully removed the possession, following which the elder sister recovered.

After giving this history I have then asked the professionals to whom I am making the presentation to give me their formulation (a summary of the relevant facts and a conclusion as to what they think is happening) based on this history as it is. I have found the responses that the professionals give interesting in three ways.

First, those with a different professional training tend to concentrate on different aspects of the history in their formulation. Thus, the psychiatrists seem to be interested in the phenomenology (a way of symptom collection for psychiatrists based on categorizing the patient's reported experiences and observed behaviour into symptom categories, for example the whisperings in the ear can be categorized as an auditory hallucination) and in their conclusions have tended to try and work out what they believe are the relevant diagnoses. Psychotherapists have been much more interested in the personal aspects of the history as well as my experience and the feelings provoked in me by being with 'A'. Their conclusions have tended to concentrate on the possible intrapersonal experiences going on in this young boy's mind, particularly at an unconscious level. Family therapists have tended to be most interested in context, wanting to know more about the experience of migration under traumatic circumstances, arriving in a new culture and 'A's' apparent sense of a lack of belonging in his peer group. Thus their conclusions have tended to concentrate more on these interpersonal aspects of the history. This is, of course, a generalization and it should be noted that there is also a considerable crossover between different professional groups' approaches. What I have been noting, however, is the general trends in different professional groups' responses. This is perhaps not surprising, given that the different trainings emphasize and are interested in these different aspects. I do think this is worthy of note because I am here presenting an identical history and this identical history is, to a significant degree, stimulating different thought processes in different professional groups. In real-life clinical situations this means that the type of questions, the style of interview, the sort of conclusions and action taken by the interviewer will vary to a significant degree according to the professional training (for exactly the same presentation). In my experience of working in different child psychiatric clinics there is no foolproof way of deciding what case is suitable for what professional. It is largely a matter of hierarchy, history and tradition, as well as complicated internal dynamics, that leads to the decisions about what type of professional will carry out which assessment.

Second, there appears to be a lack of consensus, certainly on first presentation within each professional group. I have been particularly interested in the psychiatrists' responses, as of course this is my main professional background. I have noted down the range of diagnoses being mentioned following presentation of this history. These have included early schizophrenia, manic depression, reactive depression, hysterical conversion, generalized anxiety, post-traumatic stress disorder, victim of abuse, drug-induced psychosis and paranoid psychosis. What is interesting to me is that the psychiatrists invariably followed the diagnosis route as their pathway to understanding the situation and yet that framework produced such a huge variety of possible conclusions. There wasn't even unanimous agreement as to whether this boy was psychotic (had lost touch with reality) or not. To me this echoes in microform the whole history of psychiatry's attempt to categorize the so-called 'culture-bound syndromes'.

The third response of professionals is discussed later in the chapter, see p. 41.

The problem of culture

The 'culture-bound syndromes' have been problematic for psychiatry, causing all sorts of confusion for the western-trained psychiatrist's attempt to find a neat slot into which presentations, found only in specific cultural groups, could fit within our existing psychiatric classifications.

In the early part of the last century, one of the founding fathers of western psychiatry first formulated the standard approach that modern western psychiatry takes towards understanding cross-cultural differences in symptom presentation. Kraepelin (1913) observed that patients in mental hospitals in Java were seldom depressed, and that when they were depressed, rarely felt sinful. Kraepelin, taking his native German patients as the norm against which to analyse these differences, concluded that these and other cross-cultural differences were likely caused by factors such as heredity, prenatal damage and early life illness (Kraepelin, 1920). In his analyses Kraepelin chose to ignore culture as a significant influence in favour of the idea that these presentations have universal biological origins.

This set the scene for subsequent western psychiatric analyses of presentations found in (culturally) non-western populations. Two dominant themes emerge from this transcultural psychiatric literature. First is the search for the universal at the expense of interest in cultural difference. Second is the covert assumption that western culture is the norm against which other cultures can be compared. Thus much of the mainstream transcultural psychiatry of the last century was taken up with the effort to show how these so-called 'culture-bound syndromes' could be fitted into existing psychiatric nosology.

Take, for example, the condition known as 'latah'. This condition is found mainly in south-east Asian women, with the afflicted person copying the movements or speech of other people. In a study of latah, where psychiatrists carried out psychiatric interviews of sufferers (Chiu et al., 1972), they concluded that some had no psychiatric disorder, some had depressive disorders, some hysterical neurosis, some an adjustment reaction and some schizophrenia. The researchers must have gone through an interesting process of reassessing the importance and weight given to particular experiences and behaviours to move the classification out of one system (where they are locally classified as having latah) to another (where they are classified as having depression, hysteria, schizophrenia and so on). In contrast to this approach where latah is not being conceptualized as a syndrome itself, psychiatrists have also approached latah as if it has a one-to-one correspondence with an existing psychiatric syndrome. Thus latah has been considered as an early form of schizophrenia (Chapman, 1966); a depressive state (Kenny, 1978); a culture-free physiological hyperstartle response (Simons, 1980); a female attention-seeking response (Chiu *et al.*, 1972); a toxic confusional state (Carluccio *et al.*, 1964); a form of Gilles de la Tourette syndrome (Gilles de la Tourette, 1885) and a stereotyped movement disorder (Prince and Tcheng-Laroche, 1987).

Western psychiatrists have struggled to know how or where to conceptualize such culture-bound syndromes as belonging. The main thrust seems to be that of using white western culture and its concepts as the norm against which these 'exotic' syndromes should be compared (Fernando, 1988). As Littlewood (1986) points out, culture-bound syndromes have mainly been regarded by western psychiatry, not as 'real' entities, but as local erroneous conceptualizations that shape universal forms of reaction. The validity of this approach is highly questionable. The underlying supposition seems to be that an interpretation of these syndromes in terms of western psychiatric concepts is an advance on a purely culture-bound interpretation. Such a culture-blind approach has only added to the difficulty western psychiatry has with this issue. Thus it is not clear in the existing framework for classification whether culture-bound syndromes should have a special place, a category of their own, or whether they should essentially be ignored and viewed as a cultural envelope for a condition that is already established and described in the existing psychiatric classification (Prince and Tcheng-Laroche, 1987). Berrios and Morley (1984) suggest that culture-bound syndromes should be viewed as specific niches in which psychotherapeutic routines that are socially meaningful can be activated. Prince and Tcheng-Laroche (1987: 4) conceptualize them as 'a collection of signs and symptoms (excluding notions of cause) which is restricted to a limited number of cultures, primarily by means of certain of their psychosocial features'. Leff (1988: 22) views them as 'some characteristic of humankind that might otherwise remain ignored, unexpressed or even buried in the depths of the unconscious and is brought out into overt expression by a particular culture in which it fulfils a function for the individual or his social group'. Some can't even be bothered to think about them or grapple with the challenge they present to western psychiatry, 'The more culture bound they are, the less interest they can have for psychiatry and the more for social anthropology. They are better regarded as evidence of the pathoplastic effect of culture . . . fuller examination always reveals similarities with western psychiatric concepts' (Bebbington, 1997: 480). So here he's telling us that culture-bound syndromes have little to do with psychiatry, but actually they are no different to western psychiatric concepts. What a muddle!

What hasn't been borne in mind in these attempts to think western about non-western expressions of 'something being wrong', is that psychiatric categories were developed with reference to a particular cultural group. When applied to other cultural groups our concepts may well lack coherence or credibility (Kleinman, 1987). Kleinman (1977) is particularly critical of mainstream psychiatry's assumption that deviance can be studied in different societies as if it is independent of specific cultural norms and local patterns of normative behaviour. A psychiatrist colleague of mine who trained and first practised in India before coming to the UK, commented on how much easier diagnosis became once she began practising in the UK, 'I couldn't believe it, patients told me their diagnosis, they told me they were depressed'. In India it was very rare for a patient to present complaining of depression.

Many key western psychiatric symptoms refer to conceptual constructs influenced by western philosophical ideas. These symptoms may be absent, nonsensical or have entirely different meanings in cultures where different philosophical traditions have been influential (Krause, 1989). There are few societies in the world where depression is associated with guilt, as it often is in the predominatly Jewish and Christian west (Jackson, 1985). Yet, having feelings of guilt is one of the cornerstone symptoms for the psychiatric diagnosis of depression, and it appears in most psychiatric questionnaires that screen for depression. Hopelessness is another key symptom in diagnosing depression and is one of the main features described by women in central London who complain of depression (Brown and Harris, 1978). Yet symptoms like guilt and hopelessness are unlikely to be relevant for Buddhists in Sri Lanka for whom taking pleasure from things in the world of social relationships is the basis of suffering. A wilful hopelessness and dysphoria, on the other hand, can be the first step on the road to salvation for this group (Obeyesekere, 1985). For Shiite Muslims in Iran, grief is a religious experience and the ability to experience this fully is a measure of a person's depth and level of understanding (Kleinman and Good, 1985). In such communities, as for many Hindus in India (Chakraborty and Sandel, 1984) and Muslims in Britain (Currer, 1986), the feeling of 'hope for ones self' is negatively valued and something which the person may feel they have little autonomy over in any case.

The classification and methodology in child psychiatry has been spawned from the same system. First a gender cleavage took place. In a famous, apparently ground-breaking study (Rutter *et al.*, 1970a, 1970b), in which all 8- to 11-year-old children on the Isle of Wight were screened for 'psychiatric disorder', the two groupings of emotional/internalizing and conduct/externalizing accounted for 96 per cent of all 'disordered' children. This finding contributed towards the two major western psychiatric classificatory systems, the *International Classification of Diseases* and the *Diagnostic and Statistical Manual of Mental Disorders*. These systems, influenced by the Isle of Wight study and similar methods of screening such as the child behaviour checklist (Achenbach and Edelbrock, 1978), developed classification of psychiatric disorder in childhood using an internalizing/ externalizing split. Two diagnostic categories developed, conduct disorder (naughty boys) and emotional disorder (unhappy girls). These two categories reflect the predominant male way of externalizing as opposed to the predominant female way of internalizing. Thus child psychiatry had its first simplistic system dominated by a primitive dualism characteristic of western philosophy. This then formed the blueprint from which to develop apparently more elaborate diagnostic categories. With money to be made and research grants up for grabs a medical 'sharpening up' took place. Where a disorder couldn't be medicalized then at least it could become syndromized. Once problems were medicalized, then the doors opened in psychiatric culture as with many other aspects of modern culture, and children were treated as if they were miniature adults. Now, apparently, children suffer with depression, obsessive compulsive disorder, manic-depression and so on, at far more crippling rates than we had imagined, with about 20 per cent of children and adolescents having a psychiatric disorder at any one point in time (Cohen *et al.*, 1993; McGee *et al.*, 1990; Offord *et al.*, 1987), and requiring far higher numbers and doses of drugs than we had imagined. The pharmaceutical industry has been very happy indeed about these developments. As in adult psychiatry the problem of culture has been tackled by avoiding it. As in adult psychiatry the concepts that have been developed by western child psychiatrists are viewed as the normal, correct way to interpret all manner of childhood and adolescent problems in all manner of cultural groups.

Take, for example, one of the dominant books used for training child psychiatrists *Child Psychiatry – A Developmental Approach* (Graham, 1986). In Chapter 1, *An Overview*, Dr Graham is already demonstrating the complete inability of child psychiatric literature to engage in anything other than racist stereotypes for dealing with cultural difference. It is also built on the desire to see the existing western child-psychiatric framework as the best and correct system for universal classification. Thus Graham concludes that existing evidence demonstrates that about one in five children show a significant psychological/psychiatric problem in any one year and that these rates are similar in different ethnic minority groups. Then comes the stereotyping. In discussing cognitive development and educational attainment of Asian children in the UK, Graham considers that the educational attainment of this group is higher because they have a higher proportion of more affluent self-employed or professional parents. Asians are lumped together as a group by this racist stereotyping of Asians as affluent. There is no mention of different Asian back-grounds (Bangladeshi immigrants are among the poorest in the UK), the influence of different family values and forms, or the daily experience of racism that many have to endure. Instead the minority from the immigrant Asian community who are affluent is highlighted as the sole reason for one difference amongst a cultural sub-group of children in the UK. Further on, in discussing 'West Indian children' in the UK (note he defines this group in a way that excludes them from being British), he states 'A relative lack of toys and opportunity for parent–child interaction sometimes makes the early years of the child's life relatively unstimulated' (Graham, 1986: 7). This insulting statement about the parenting abilities of West Indian origin parents is made without any reference to the evidence for this. And this pretty much concludes the book's reference to the influence of culture.

My personal experience that culture as a dimension is ignored in favour of the idea that we already know the universally valid child-psychiatric syndromes, was further confirmed when I searched through the last 5-years' worth of articles from the two leading mainstream academic child-psychiatry journals.

First the *Journal of the American Academy of Child and Adolescent Psychiatry*. I looked at all copies of this journal printed between October 1996 and October 2001 (a total of 60 issues, each containing 15 to 20 articles). In the few articles that referred to children from non-western cultures, I read about attention deficit hyperactivity disorder in Ukrainian schoolchildren, Tourette's syndrome in Costa Rica, parent management training in China and the effects of war on Cambodian children. These few cross-cultural papers used western-developed questionnaires (with no discussion about the validity of these questionnaires other than in their linguistic translation). All used western child-psychiatric concepts to analyse the results. None discussed the question of cultural influences in anything more than a vague superficial manner. Livingston's paper 'Cultural issues in the diagnosis and treatment of Attention Deficit Hyperactivity Disorder' (Livingston, 1999), illustrates how culture is viewed through this psychiatric lens. This paper describes five case histories of American ethnic-minority children where the author felt that cultural issues obscured diagnosis and treatment. The general thrust of the paper is that cultural factors can result in a failure to diagnose and adequately treat attention deficit hyperactivity disorder (ADHD). The paper implicitly accepts that the western child psychiatric label of ADHD is cross-culturally valid and there is no attempt to discuss its cultural appropriateness. Instead, the analyses of cultural factors take up superficial, stereotyped issues with the doctor 'educating' these families about this 'medical' disorder and its treatment in order to resolve these dilemmas. For example, with one Muslim family it is suggested that during the fasting month of Ramadan doses of medication may need to be altered or a longer-acting drug given in the morning. It is suggested that higher doses of medication may need to be given for children whose cultures 'prize educational achievement'. When a black mother raises her concern that her son's teacher has suggested that her son has ADHD, because, as the mother sees it, there is a problem of 'an inexperienced white teacher who wants to drug children into compliance', rather than legitimizing that in a racist society such concerns may be valid, the author chooses to view this as a cultural issue that can be resolved by educating the parent. This he does by siding with the teacher's opinion and her child is given medication. This, in my opinion, is the attitude and practice of a colonizer.

The other journal I looked at was the *Journal of Child Psychology and Psychiatry*. I looked through all the issues between September 1996 and September 2001 (48 issues each with 10 to 15 articles). The papers in this journal are so densely written and full of statistical mystification and bio-babble that most are virtually unreadable. Again there were very few articles that involved any cross-cultural research and all of these used translated versions of western-developed questionnaires without discussing the cultural validity of doing this. Most authors interpreted their findings in a way that allowed them to conform to western psychiatric concepts and theories, showing little interest in indigenous beliefs and practices. In a rare exception the paper by McCarty *et al.* (1999) did discuss, in an interesting and informative manner, how different cultural beliefs and practices affect the way Thai and American young people deal with different types of stresses. In my opinion, therefore, only one article out of a total of about 1600 journal articles published over 5 years, from the two leading academic child-psychiatric journals, said anything to suggest that culture is an important dimension. None of the articles questioned the validity of the constructs and questionnaires that were used.

Thus, in child and adolescent psychiatry as in adult psychiatry, a western-developed psychiatric framework is imposed in a way that ignores and minimizes cultural variation. Such a culture-blind belief system has left psychiatry with a big headache when it comes to developing universally valid systems for categorizing mental-health problems.

Invented by doctors, psychiatry's primary mode of thinking in the complex area of human problems is the symptom-gathering approach. We gather our medical evidence (in this case symptoms, what the patient says and how she/he behaves) to arrive at our medical conclusion. To test and expand our medical hypothesis we use the language and accepted customs of medicine. Naturally, when we enter into a discussion on the evidence supporting the existence of an idea (e.g. depression, schizophrenia) within this medical framework, we have usually already left behind other frameworks for analysing and interpreting what doctors are calling depression, schizophrenia, etc., and enter into the language and thinking of the medical frame. We then select the bits of evidence that agree with, and can be fitted into, our frame and choose to ignore, minimize and/or deny the existence of those bits that threaten to upset the applecart (just as I expect I am doing in this book). After all, if your beliefs, particularly ones that are fundamental to you, fall apart, so does your world. This selective approach to interpreting the results of existing cross-cultural studies has further strengthened psychiatry's claims to have developed a universally valid system for classifying what it refers to as mental-health problems.

Framework to fit the evidence or evidence to fit the framework?

One of the most widely quoted sources of 'proof' that schizophrenia is an illness found the world over, that I recall learning about in my psychiatric training, is the international study carried out for the World Health Organization (WHO). In 1961, WHO began a study in nine countries – Britain, Columbia, Czechoslovakia, Denmark, Taiwan, India, Nigeria, the Soviet Union and the US. This project set out to discover if schizophrenia could be diagnosed according to standardized criteria in all nine countries and if so with what rate of incidence. The study concluded that in all nine countries, there was a group of patients who presented with similar sets of symptoms that fitted the criteria for schizophrenia and at a similar rate of incidence, apart from two countries, the Soviet Union and the US, which both had higher rates of incidence. The higher rates in these two countries was, we were told, put down to differences in the way the category of schizophrenia was defined (standardized? criteria?) in these two countries and therefore unlikely to represent a 'true' higher rate. The study concluded that schizophrenia must therefore be a universal condition, as it can be found in all social and cultural settings with a similar rate of occurrence, a pattern which suggests that schizophrenia is a biological condition (World Health Organization 1973, 1979). This is what I was taught. This was the party line if you wished to pass your professional exams and progress in your career.

All I was told about in my training turned out to be just a few of the pieces of the jigsaw. The rest seemed to go missing or was ignored. It was irrelevant, no need to muddy the picture after all. First, most of the psychiatric patients who presented at the different clinical centres had to be excluded since they did not fit the criteria. This suggested the possibility that what the study had accomplished was to use a template that effectively stamped out a pattern of complaints that would have produced a more heterogeneous sample. In other words the selection criteria ensured that a similar group of patients would be selected. Second, despite this homogenizing-template approach, there were still important cross-cultural divergences that were ignored (such as the predominance of different symptom profiles in different centres) in favour of highlighting similarities. Third, the logic behind the conclusion that similar prevalence rates means a biological illness is flawed. Very few other medical, biological illnesses have similar prevalence rates across diverse social and cultural groupings. In fact it is the reverse of the argument of evolutionary biologists who argue that biology is a major source of variation causing great diversity in species worldwide (Mayr, 1981). Fourth, patients in the study may not have come from as widely differing cultural belief systems as the investigators would like to believe, coming as they did from locations near established university hospitals where 'westernization' was more likely to take place. Fifth, the psychiatrists in this project had studied in the same psychiatric traditions (often at the same universities) and were thus more likely to have fitted any, in their eyes, abnormal behaviour into their preferred psychiatric framework. They may well have minimized the perceived importance of other large areas of difference, for example the content of the diagnosed patient's utterances (Littlewood and Lipsedge, 1989). It is not surprising that the study found what it set out to find.

Beyond the confines of this study further evidence that is apparently best ignored is forthcoming. There are massive regional variations in the rates of diagnosis of schizophrenia. The highest rates of diagnosis are found among West Indians in Britain, on the west coast of Ireland, among Croatians on the Dalmatian coast, in French-Canadians, in Native Americans, in Australian Aborigines and New Zealand Maori (colonized minorities?) (Littlewood, 1999). Societies with little westernization appear in some studies to have much lower rates of diagnosable schizophrenia and for those diagnosed a much better prognosis (Torrey *et al.*, 1974; Nandi, 1980; Kleinman, 1996).

Perhaps the most serious blow to the WHO study was its own follow up of the original sample 2 years later (Sartorius *et al.*, 1977, 1986). Patients in Europe and the US were nearly three times more likely to be regarded as actively 'ill' 2 years on, than were patients from developing countries, this despite patients in western countries receiving more thorough psychiatric treatment and more medication than their counterparts in the underdeveloped areas of the world. Of course this finding, and the many other similar ones concerning outcome in developing countries, are often explained away by the mainstream campaigners, as being to do with methodological problems in the study and not a 'true' finding. It would seem that the study, having imposed a western-disease-derived concept, in finding that western medical treatment does not contribute to a favourable outcome, has raised questions about the very concept of schizophrenia and the conclusion that this is a biological condition. This must be a hard pill to swallow for the investigators. No wonder the authors of the ambitious *Determinants of Outcome* study (Sartorius *et al.*, 1997, 1986) chose in their discussion to be silent on the most important point they found, that is the better outcome of the poorly treated (by western medical standards) group (Kleinman, 1988). Why was I not taught this early on? The original conclusions are unsustainable. There is really little evidence to suggest that what was being called schizophrenia in the original WHO study, was in fact the same 'illness' being discovered universally by those great pioneering psychiatrists. The study raised more serious questions about this western idea than it did answers.

Thus the concepts born out of the dominant systems for classifying what psychiatrists call 'mental disorders' are based on a selective interpretation of evidence to allow the evidence to fit the framework. The framework is theoretically derived, contains unproven assumptions about aaetiology and is born out of consensus of a body of powerful (culturally) western psychiatrists. It assumes that its concepts represent a kind of universal truth about mental disorders. It assumes that it has discovered the norm, against which presentations of 'something wrong' not recognized in western culture, can be understood. Not surprisingly child psychiatrists too have shown themselves to be better at relying on the consensus of the powerful to back up their ideas, than on the analysis of evidence. Where evidence is collected it is analysed in a way that allows it to fit into the mainstream western psychiatric framework. Child psychiatrists also assume they have discovered a universal, scientific truth about the disorders they diagnose and harbour the same implicit assumptions about aaetiology in their diagnoses.

In an authoritative review of the existing evidence behind the current classifications used in child and adolescent psychiatry, Cantwell and Rutter conclude 'it is clearly evident that differentiation between the main diagnostic categories has major clinical meaning already' (1994: 11). Yet earlier in this review the high comorbidity (a child having more than one diagnosis) in child psychiatry (Caron and Rutter, 1991) was mentioned and they suggested that this high degree of overlap between child psychiatric syndromes 'may reflect inadequate conceptualization of the disorders' (Cartwell and Rutter, 1994: 6). The article reviews all the possible ways in which the categories used in child psychiatry could be shown to have a scientific basis. Aaetiology, statistical grouping of symptoms, epidemiological data, long-term course, genetic findings, psychosocial risk factors, neuropsychological patterns, biological investigations and drug response, are all suggested to have been of little help in developing diagnostic specificity. Yet the authors still concluded that child-psychiatric diagnostic categories had major clinical meaning. Predictably there was no mention of cultural issues or cross-cultural validity of the concepts used. Child-psychiatric classification is based on the consensus of a powerful group of western-trained psychiatrists. My main criticism is that this fact is not made more explicit. The classification system we use is based on opinion not fact. We do not know if we are diagnosing naturally occurring 'real' entities or imposing our own prejudiced perceptions. We know that those opinions that have been given the most weight in developing this consensus system are culturally western in their outlook. Their attitudes and value judgements are likely to reflect the racist and colonial mentality of the society out of which their profession came into being (Fernando, 1988).

Back to the case study

For the psychiatrists to verify their proposed diagnosis for the boy 'A', they suggested they needed further information, observation, etc. None of them were able to suggest a single physical test that would reflect some material reality in this boy's body (such as an x-ray, brain scan or chemical in the blood) that could substantiate their proposed diagnosis. That's because there isn't any. Physical tests we ask for in child psychiatry are usually to do with excluding known physical causes. Unlike the rest of medicine, in psychiatry there is no way of reinforcing a subjective opinion about diagnosis with material evidence. Diagnosis, therefore, rests on subjective theory driven assumptions rather than on what one might call hard factual medicine. It is therefore also not surprising that the same confusion concerning classification appears in clinical practice even where the cultural differences could be said to be less than in this example (the boy 'A'). During my time doing adult psychiatric training, the repeated experience with patients who had chronic mental-health problems and several admissions to hospital was that their diagnosis would have changed at least once, but more often several times, during that time. I also recall, during one placement in the psychiatry of old age, I worked on a ward where many of the patients had been long-term psychiatric patients, sometimes over the previous 50 years or more. Their records made fascinating reading. They too had many different diagnoses applied to them at different stages in their hospital career. Some had originally been admitted with a diagnosis of moral insanity after becoming pregnant out of wedlock. This made me wonder what will happen to our current psychiatric classification. How long before most of the categories we use today become outdated?

The confusion doesn't stop there. Different countries developed different diagnostic frameworks, the most well known currently being the *International Classification of Diseases* (ICD, published by the World Health Organization) and the *Diagnostic and Statistical Manual of Mental Disorders* (DSM, published by the American Psychiatric Association). But there are other systems. For example the system that arose in France and is still used in France and many African countries. Then there is the psychiatric classification system that developed in eastern Europe during the cold war years. Clinicians who put their faith in those systems that owe their origins to modernist western culture have been quick to criticize the practice of psychiatry in eastern Europe as being driven by political and social motives (Bloch and Reddaway, 1977; Kiev, 1968). They accuse eastern European psychiatry of inappropriately labelling political dissidents as mentally ill and incarcerating them in psychiatric hospitals (more on this in Chapter 6). What has not been available to a similar analysis by those critics is how much our own diagnostic criteria are also a product of particular political and social circumstances. Two brief examples that speak for themselves will suffice. First, the gross over representation of lower social classes in psychiatric hospitals (Dunham, 1964; Bebbington et al., 1981). Second, the consistent evidence that patients of African or Caribbean origin living in the UK (mainly second generation) are grossly over represented in admissions to psychiatric beds (Dean et al., 1981; Bhugra et al., 1977). In admissions to secure psychiatric settings (Cope, 1989; Coid et al., 2000), they are more likely to be subject to compulsory psychiatric treatment (Browne, 1990) and are more likely to be referred by police for urgent psychiatric assessments (Bean et al., 1991).

Back to the professionals' responses to my case presentation (see p. 32).

At the end of my presentation of the case of the boy 'A' the third, and for me the most interesting, feature of the responses that I have received to date, is that I have not come across a western-trained professional who has either suggested that this patient may be possessed, or who has been interested in this possibility, which, after all, is the boy's own (and possibly his family's own) explanation for his predicament. Naturally, I accept that, putting it in research terminology, my sample of professionals is a necessarily limited and statistically small one. My impression is that the majority of western-trained professionals of all persuasions would only be interested in the boy's and his family's own explanation(s) in a negative way, i.e. they have no validity. There seems to be a strongly held belief amongst the professional groups this case history has been presented to, that the explanation of being possessed by a djinn is at best misguided, at worst a potentially harmful superstition or an excuse to cover up more serious problems (e.g. child abuse).

Yet, I have to ask this question, can any of us armed with our professional explanations provide any greater material evidence to suggest that our explanations are closer to the ultimate truth about this situation than those who are armed with the explanation that this is the result of a supernatural possession by a djinn? Do we not go through exactly the same process to arrive at a conclusion as the imam does when diagnosing a state of possession by a djinn? Each of us concentrates on those aspects of the presenting picture that, according to our interpretive framework, are relevant to reach our conclusions. Our conclusions are then different according to the framework that we have been using. The same picture looks different through different lenses. Neither the professional nor the imam has access to any material findings or hard facts to support their conclusions.

Then one day, during a home visit to a client, I truly risked suspending my professional beliefs. I sat in the room of a 16-year-old boy who (together with his family) believed he was possessed. I had already learned that djinns prey on the vulnerable and can cross from one human to another. For a short time, towards the end of the session, I let myself believe that this boy was possessed. I became frightened. I knew very little about djinns, how to work when they're around and how to protect myself against them. I was walking into the unknown. Was that grimace on his face the work of the djinn? How much control does he have? How much of what I was told today was the djinn speaking? Was that shiver I felt inside me the djinn getting into me? I left with a headache which stayed with me for the rest of that day. Was that a sign that the djinn was in me? That night I had a vivid dream. I had come home to find my house on fire, with massive hot flames lighting up the night sky. The next day I had to get on with work and family and forgot the events of the previous day and life carried on. Then a couple of months later a Muslim scholar told me that djinns are often symbolized by fire. I have no explanation for the events of that strange day when I stepped completely out of my mental-health professional strait-jacket.

Psychiatry is based on faith

In the paragraphs above I am trying to point out some essential similarities in the processes that take place within the interviewer when trying to understand a clinical picture. Clinical pictures are filtered through pre-existing frameworks that channel the interviewer's thinking in a particular direction, leading to a particular conclusion. These conclusions cannot, in the current state of knowledge, represent any ultimate truth as they cannot be confirmed or refuted by verifiable material facts. Yet the majority of professionals I meet seem to be convinced that their framework is dealing with some sort of ultimate truth. Thus, the psychiatrist who is diagnosing a major mental illness believes very strongly that he has diagnosed a biological form of disease to the brain and will think and act in a way that corresponds to that conclusion. The family therapist may find her/himself evaluating the context, for example the family, according to some pre-existing normative assumptions about family functioning, and, from their analysis of the clinical picture, reach similarly strongly held conclusions about an abnormality in the patterns of functioning. The psychotherapist will come armed with assumptions concerning the basis for normality and development of internal mental life. The imam will be taking their own assumptions concerning spiritual life and supernatural forces to assess the clinical picture.

What is it that keeps people believing in the truth of their way of understanding the same picture when there is no way of proving this? I think that in the absence of proof we use faith to sustain our belief in something. We then sift through the evidence in a selective way to reinforce our faith and discredit those we feel are non-believers.

In this chapter I have attempted to deconstruct professional models and suggest that they have a lot more to do with human constructs and processes than hard science. I have also suggested that one of the factors that keeps practitioners believing in the models that they adopt has something to do with what I am calling faith feelings. This might seem a little bit paradoxical for practitioners who have been trained in modernist, western approaches, particularly as these approaches have often tried to set themselves apart from religious and faith practices, by suggesting that their methodologies and insights are somehow more progressive, enlightened and scientific. Arrogant superiority and contempt for other cultures, particularly those more dominated by supernatural explanations of their world, permeates western mental-health culture at every level. As Fernando (1988) has shown, eminent and influential psychiatrists have in the past and present carried on this shameful tradition. As psychiatry flourished, the culturally predominant racist ideas were incorporated into its theories. This has included views about the (alleged) inferiority of black people with regard to their brain size (Bean, 1906), psychological maturity (Hall, 1904) and emotional functioning (Jung, 1930). These ideas became deeply embedded within western psychiatric thinking with the result that 'coloured' people and people from cultures different to our own came to be thought of as inferior. References to this apparent inferiority are in abundance and include comments about personality deviance (Kardiner and Ovesey, 1951), brain quality (Carothers, 1951), low intelligence (Jensen, 1969), living in 'primitive cultures' (e.g. Bebbington, 1978), coping by 'cheery denial' (Bebbington *et al.*, 1981) and lacking psychological or emotional sophistication (e.g. Leff, 1973).

Yet this is all so unnecessary. There is nothing shameful about having faith, about needing to believe. It is essentially very human. Feelings of faith can help to keep one's world together, help it to make sense, and for many faith falling apart is like the world falling apart. I have come across many clients for whom religion has become much more central following a difficult experience in their lives, for example refugees fleeing from war, torture and other terrifying life events. Religion provides some sense of orientation, continuity and a map from which to continue to structure one's life and make sense of what is happening. I think a very similar process goes on for a professional. If a long-held belief in the correctness of a professional's most trusted model begins to fall apart, a similar feeling of disorientation and a falling apart of the professional world occurs with the loss of a sense of identity and professional self-esteem. Of course there is large variation between practitioners as to the extent and strength with which they hold their beliefs, with some who could be described as fundamentalist believers in their professional model and others who could be described as being more agnostic, operating in between models. There are even those who could be described as being atheist who may completely reject the model they were trained in. Freud, though originally very critical of the role of faith in people's lives (Freud, 1913), later saw much value in religion, seeming to recognize that beliefs and values are necessary and that science is unlikely to attain 'the desired primacy of intelligence over the life of the instincts. This is surely an illusion. In this decisive respect human nature is hardly likely to change.' (Freud, 1927: 235).

When it comes to the process of questioning the assumptions held by different theoretical models and their relative usefulness, it is also important to understand something of the cultural origins of these models. The dominant professional models that us practitioners use are derived from modern, western culture. Dominant psychiatric models have a history based within the development of western medical science. Those fundamentalist practitioners of disease-model-based psychiatry spend their time emphasizing this paradigm and wax lyrical on the importance of the randomized controlled trial as the gold standard by which truths are generated. Those theories, ideas or reflections that do not involve this gold standard are usually rejected as unproven. Thus, those ideas that are easier to investigate, using the randomized controlled trial (e.g. response to medication), tend to achieve a high status within this modernist religion. The more psychological paradigms such as psychoanalysis, systemic theory, cognitive and behavioural theory, construct a view about human relationships and how they go wrong that is also clearly derived from modern, western, cultural preoccupations (Pilgrim, 1997). All these systems rely on an idea. The idea is all too often confused with the thing itself. The randomized controlled trial investigates an idea, not a known disease state. There is only a human construct in the starting block; the science can therefore never really get off the starting line here. What we have is faith. Why are we so afraid to admit this? After all science is the dominant western cultural method used for explaining and understanding the world around us and our place in it, it is the faith filter for our cosmology.

Chapter 4

Reversing the form/content argument

Psychiatry has argued that patterns of mental distress or illness have a definable core (defined by orthodox psychiatry as the form) which it regards as universal and whose presentation (defined by orthodox psychiatry as the content) is shaped by a cultural envelope. In this chapter I will argue that the opposite way of conceptualizing form and content is more accurate and more revealing. I will argue that it is the different possible interpretations of the same presentation that make up the content (of the attempt to understand that presentation). This content is in turn shaped by the cultural model (the form) being used as the framework for defining the meaning of that presentation.

The psychiatric form/content argument

If you agreed with my last chapter where I suggested that any system used to arrive at an understanding of somebody's mental-health problems requires a certain degree of faith on the part of the practitioner, then I think it is easy to follow how this second proposition derives from the first one.

Psychiatry has traditionally treated, and to this very day continues to treat, culture as a thin veneer that colours the mental-health presentations of different individuals and that underneath this thin veneer so-called mental illnesses and disorders are essentially the same. Furthermore, it is argued that psychiatry works from and uses scientifically generated knowledge that has been validated across cultures. The arguments within psychiatry tend to take place around how to define these categories and sub-categories, rather than the wholesale questioning of the scientific validity of these categories. As explored in the last chapter, there are assumptions of superiority and infallibility that go along with a strong conviction or faith and a position of high power and status. The position of power that psychiatrists occupy ensures that their sense of infallibility remains difficult to shift. Those psychiatrists who have challenged the assumptions underlying what is essentially a social construct have often been ostracized and marginalized. Anybody who, like myself, has had some experience of working as a psychiatrist with non-establishment views will know very well how difficult it is to survive such an environment without compromising your own sanity and chances of progression in your career (see Chapters 1 and 5).

Psychiatric training in the UK is about learning the psychiatric belief system with the underlying assumption that psychiatric disorders occur in a similar manner worldwide, in accordance with the definitions taught and with culture being a thin veneer that sometimes shapes the content of whatever disorder we discover. In this system it is assumed that there is such an illness as schizophrenia (the form) and that the basic symptoms of schizophrenia, such as delusions, hallucinations and nonsensical speech, are the same all over the world. It is assumed that schizophrenia is a biologically based disease and it is this disease that causes the structure of, say, a delusional thought process. It is then claimed that what can vary is the cultural influence on these symptoms (in other words content). Thus, it is argued that in certain parts of the world you may have delusions that the CIA is after you, in others the delusion may be of the devil trying to kill you.

This is the basic traditional psychiatric form/content argument. There are universal psychiatric categories (form), shaped by local environmental factors (content). People's belief systems, lifestyle, life circumstances and so on are treated as having a minor influence and influence only how these underlying diseases express themselves. All being well, the psychiatrist graduates from her/his training with the belief that she/he is equipped to recognize and accurately categorize mental illnesses through a method of symptom collecting that will hold good with clients from all backgrounds, providing the psychiatrist remembers that they only need understand that culture will shape how their client expresses the symptoms and not the symptoms themselves.

For example, psychiatric researchers repeatedly claim that bodily complaints predominate over psychological complaints in depressive disorders among members of non-western societies, ethnic minorities and less-educated members of the lower socio-economic classes (Leff, 1981; Kirmayer, 1984). This finding, skewed as it is by a western psychiatric concept, is interpreted as meaning that the biology of depression is universal, with cultural factors influencing how this disease is expressed. It is usually suggested that bodily complaints come to 'mask' the 'real' psychiatric disease, because of the lack of psychological sophistication within the sufferer (Leff, 1973). In this model diagnosis becomes a reductionistic exercise whereby the psychiatrist carefully picks out the cultural colouring to reveal the underlying disease. Viewing the evidence using different theoretical frameworks leads to very different conclusions, not only about the meaning of the symptoms, patterns of health-seeking behaviour and treatment response, but about the very existence of a disease called depression.

As many anthropologically informed authors have suggested, the mental state of 'depression' cannot be viewed separately from the local cultural meanings it contains (Kleinman and Good, 1985). Thus, among some South Pacific island communities depression is not seen as the opposite of happiness (Lutz, 1985). The Kaluli in Papua New Guinea do not recognize or have a label for depression (Schieffelin, 1985). Buddhists in Sri Lanka positively value what western culture calls depression, believing that pleasurable attachments to people and things are the roots of all suffering and that the recognition of the ultimate hopelessness of existence makes transcendence possible (Obeyesekere, 1985). Indeed the western psychiatric concept of depression is highly culturally embedded, having developed from various explanatory systems used in western culture including moral and religious systems, before becoming a medicopsychological label (Jackson, 1985). Lutz (1985) argues that the concept of depression has been influenced by philosophical ideas (such as the mind–body dichotomy) taken from the west's cultural tradition, which is inevitably ethnocentric in its thinking. As White and Marsella (1982) point out, people in most cultures talk about interactions between body and consciousness; it is only when a sharp distinction between the two systems is set up (as in western psychiatric mind–body dualism) that the idea of psychosomatic illness or symptoms becomes necessary.

Taking one culture's diagnostic categories and applying it to another where these categories may lack coherence is a category fallacy (Kleinman, 1977). Obeyesekere (1985) offers a telling example. Suppose, he suggests, a south Asian psychiatrist working in an area where semen-loss syndromes are common, travelled to the US, where these syndromes have neither professional nor popular coherence. Let us imagine that this south Asian psychiatrist has first operationalized (research jargon meaning that numbers, frequency and duration of symptoms needed for a diagnosis have been defined) the category of 'semen loss', produced a psychiatric interview schedule and translated this into English. A group of American psychiatrists were then trained to use this schedule and were shown to have a high level of consistency in their diagnosis. Using this schedule, prevalence of 'semen-loss syndrome' in the US could be discovered. To a western psychiatrist the idea of diagnosing 'semen-loss syndrome' would seem completely foolish in a society that doesn't recognize 'semen loss' as a common complaint. Yet this is precisely what much cross-cultural psychiatric research has been doing. Western psychiatrists take western concepts to investigate other cultures. Where cross-cultural differences emerge these are bulldozed to fit into the existing western psychiatric framework. 'We know the truth' is what these psychiatrists are saying. Like the missionaries they see their task as freeing the people from their erroneous cultural superstitions.

In this system cultural sensitivity means providing kosher food and an occasional interpreter. Because this basic philosophy underpins most in-patient and out-patient services I have worked in, the majority are, I believe, culturally insensitive, giving little room for the development of a service that truly accommodates other belief systems. This culture-thin framework is the basis of current psychiatric teaching in adult and child psychiatry. This model is then exported worldwide.

To illustrate just how culture thin the psychiatric approach is, I've looked at the perceived role of culture in recommended training textbooks for general psychiatry and then child and adolescent psychiatry.

The main large textbook I used for learning and revising when I took my final professional exams in order to become a member of the Royal College of Psychiatrists, was *The Oxford Textbook of Psychiatry* second edition (Gelder *et al.*, 1989). References in this book to culture and belief systems are so few and far between that they can be easily summarized here. On page 341 there is one paragraph on 'cultural psychosis', in which it is mentioned that there is a high incidence of acute and transient psychosis in some developing countries that may be due to organic causes such as tropical infections. A little earlier in the chapter the World Health Organization's international pilot study of Schizophrenia (1973, which I discussed in the last chapter) is mentioned. Predictably the discrepancy in the rates of diagnosis between the US and the UK in this study is put down to diagnostic practices as opposed to a 'true' difference. Briefly I was encouraged, the better outcome for schizophrenia in developing countries is mentioned, only to be brought back to earth by the manner it is dealt with. Only one possible explanation for this finding is mentioned, selection bias, the argument being that those patients with a more insidious onset to their illness, who would have had a worse outcome, were probably not taken to hospital. And that's it. That's the sum total this massive training textbook has to say about culture.

Maybe the situation has changed since my general psychiatric training some 8 to 10 years ago. I decided to look at a more recent textbook also recommended for trainee psychiatrists preparing for their professional exams, *The Essentials of Postgraduate Psychiatry* third edition (Murray *et al.*, 1997). Right from the preface the tone of scientific superiority and definitive universality is set: 'psychiatric epidemiology has successfully moved from being merely descriptive to employing analytic techniques to address questions of cause . . . the antipsychiatry movement has almost disappeared' (Murray *et al.*, 1997: xxiv). Predictably then, in this book too, culture has no space. In the chapter on schizophrenia (Murray, 1997) there is not even a soundbite about the controversies, uncertainties and outcome studies in developing countries. There is a chapter on social and transcultural psychiatry (Bebbington, 1997). This chapter summarizes well the traditional modernist psychiatric approach to culture.

> The value of transcultural psychiatry lies not in its exotic appeal but in the way it throws light on general attributes of psychiatric disorder. The study of illness patterns across cultures illuminates the nature of illness in an absolute sense, by establishing the utility of identifying a common core of features and an outer margin whose characteristics are much more a cultural product.
>
> (Bebbington, 1997: 479)

Bebbington also makes a few brief remarks about culture-bound syndromes, stating that they are of little interest to psychiatry and that in any case they are always similar to other psychiatric categories (and therefore follow the same form/content rule he so clearly believes in). Bebbington shows, in my view, a typical fundamentalist approach in the brief dealing his chapter has on the question of culture. In relation to the massively inflated rates of diagnosis of schizophrenia in young African and Caribbean men he states 'The excess of cases of psychosis may be a cohort effect. One suggestion is that this might be mediated by exposure of Afro-Caribbean mothers to a novel infectious agent at the time of immigration' (Bebbington, 1997: 500). Sadly, that was all there was in this training manual.

So, to pass your Royal College of Psychiatry exams you must conform to the view that culture is an occasional irritation masking the 'real thing'. Anyone for institutional racism?

Perhaps the situation would be better in child and adolescent psychiatry. Surely those tasked with the understanding of the vital influences on and care of children growing and developing would appreciate the central importance of belief systems.

I decided to look at the textbook quoted most often during my child psychiatry training years, the massive *Child and Adolescent Psychiatry, Modern Approaches* third edition (Rutter *et al.*, 1994). Surely, in this book of over 1100 pages of dense small print in 64 different chapters, there would be plenty of examples of culture and belief systems being incorporated into psychiatric thinking. First disappointment, not one of 64 chapters had any reference in its title to culture. So off I went searching again. Here's what I found. In the chapter on psychological tests and assessments Berger (1994) raises briefly and superficially the concern that psychological tests may discriminate against certain minority groups, suggesting (with no guide on how you should do this) that assessors should have ongoing awareness of the possible influence that cultural factors may have on test results. Next, Taylor (1994), in his chapter on attention deficit and overactivity, looks at some studies that conclude that children in China and Hong Kong have a high rate of hyperactivity and poor attention, despite the observation that Chinese children appear less hyperactive and more attentive. The possible more controversial questions this finding might raise are ignored by Taylor, who instead chooses to conclude that the disparity is because of the greater importance school success has in China. In the chapter on schizophrenia and allied disorders, Taylor and Werry (1994) refer briefly to what they consider are the cultural effects on symptomatology, their arguments obviously conforming nicely to a medical form/content view. In the chapter on adolescent services, Steinberg (1994) states that the effect on services of cultural difference between staff and clientele has been relatively neglected. Having stated this point Steinberg then proceeds to neglect it.

In my opinion there were only two chapters that take the issue of culture semi-seriously, even if for just a very brief moment. In the chapter on psychiatric aspects of somatic disease and disorders, Mrazek (1994) discusses how professionals should take care when assessing patients that come from different cultures, concluding that the meaning of the somatic complaint needs to be interpreted in the light of knowledge about that culture's understanding of illness. Although this was helpful, it deserved more than a 'token' place in this chapter. In her chapter on family therapy, Gorell-Barnes (1994) emphasizes that white professionals need to recognize difference and question the assumptions of universality in their training. She also discusses the inequalities of structure and power built into the mental-health systems in the UK.

Finally, I want to mention Chapter 1 of this book which deals with classification, as this sets the gold standard for our psychiatric medical approach to the problems of children and adolescents. After briefly tracing the history of the development of classification in child and adolescent psychiatry, Cantwell and Rutter (1994) put forward, in my opinion, a very poor defence of the current system of classifying childhood psychiatric disorder. Their argument is full of political-style rambling and short on substance, for example 'During the last decade, research findings have provided an increasing body of evidence supporting the validity of some of the broad diagnostic distinctions within the field of child and adolescent disorder' (Cantwell and Rutter, 1994: 11), and 'it is clearly evident that differentiation between the main diagnostic categories has major clinical meaning already' (Cantwell and Rutter, 1994: 11), and 'the general conclusion has been that the reliability of most major psychiatric categories has been acceptably high' (Cantwell and Rutter, 1994: 13). Note the language; research findings, body of evidence, clearly evident, major clinical meaning, general conclusion, acceptably high. The language creates the dogma. It becomes propaganda and there is no need to demonstrate what you're talking about. Psychiatric classification is good and valid because we say so.

Overall then child and adolescent psychiatry teaches the same faith construct as reality. What a shame.

Reversing the form/content argument

If, as I believe, our current model of psychiatry turns out to be merely another belief system with its own ideas about how to define the problems it seeks to help and how to go about the task of helping, then the form/content argument is surely the wrong way round. It is the belief system that dictates the form through which meaning will be given to a mental-health problem with the content of that meaning being derived from the particular belief system being applied.

Let me return to the clinical example I used in Chapter 3, of the adolescent boy 'A' who believes he is possessed by a djinn, to illustrate this point. Different meanings will be given to this presentation dependent on what belief system the meaning giver (who essentially acts as a kind of cultural interpreter) uses to arrive at his or her conclusion. A traditional psychiatrist might decide this is evidence of early schizophrenia. He would have used a system of collecting symptoms and interpreting the history in a particular manner consistent with a medical model approach (form) to arrive at the conclusion that this is early schizophrenia (content). An imam will use a very different belief system and will be looking for very different phenomena and therefore be asking very different questions and collecting a different type of evidence. The imam's system will be consistent with a religious/traditional approach (form) to arrive at the conclusion that 'A' is possessed by a djinn of a particular kind (content). A family therapist may use a systemic framework to identify factors in the system that 'A' lives in (form) and come to their conclusion about what the nature of the problem is (content). A psychoanalyst may use a psychoanalytic framework to identify factors in 'A's internal world (form) to arrive at their formulation of 'A's problems (content). Each of the belief systems will generate a different sort of interview and assessment and each belief system would lead to potentially different approaches in their attempt to effect a solution to this presenting problem.

In reality of course, there are often crossovers between the conclusions of one system of thinking and that of another, although the differences become greater the more we move into systems that are unfamiliar to our cultural upbringing. The imam's system may be particularly alien to us, because as we are professionals trained in western systems of thought we are unlikely to have much knowledge or understanding of the methods used by such a system. This is likely to be experienced by us professionals as completely outside the ways of thinking that are even vaguely familiar to us. The whole concept of supernatural causes and supernatural solutions could be said to be completely alien to the western systems we are taught which rely on the idea of a scientific rationalist approach. Furthermore, as we move into belief systems that are radically different to the ones we are familiar with, even such things as placing the arguments I am putting forward onto a linear platform of a problem and solution may have little relevance to other ways of approaching life's difficulties.

Sometimes it is true to say that as a result of different beliefs we can exist in different worlds. Phrases such as 'Inshaa Allah' and 'Ibeed Allah' meaning 'God willing' and 'it is in God's hand' respectively, are used by many of my Arabic and Muslim clients (as well as in the culture I grew up in). It is part of a very different mental orientation to the future. Such a phrase is used whenever anything concerning an event in the future tense is said, reflecting a strong belief that all future events are controlled by a supreme being, that the future is predestined in some way and has a significance and meaning that only Allah (God) can understand. It sets the locus of control over life events outside the individual with the individual learning to accept and adapt to that predestiny. As I argued in the last chapter many of the symptoms that are believed to be central to western psychiatric categories (e.g. hopelessness) are not encountered in many non-western cultures, and even when they are they are given different significance.

Seeing the form/content argument in this light, unlike the traditional psychiatric approach, is what might be described as a culture-thick approach. It suggests that our interpretation of what is going on in mental-health problems is a cultural practice relying on subjective, historically, socially and politically derived systems of thought to interpret meaning (in the absence of objective material evidence).

This is a problem that psychiatry has found it impossible to escape from. Now child and adolescent psychiatry has to deal with the same problem. Unlike the rest of medicine which relies on cause-based diagnoses which can be backed with objective material evidence, such as blood tests, x-rays, scans, etc., psychiatry is limping behind trying to use the same theoretical model as the rest of medicine but without a cause-based system for diagnosis and without the existence of any objective materially based test for any of the disorders it believes exist. Psychiatry would dearly love to have a rational material basis to its theories and practices, but has yet to manage this. Instead psychiatrists have tried to replace spiritual, moral, political and folk understandings of distress and madness with the technological framework of psychopathology and neuroscience (Bracken and Thomas, 2001). The quest for a technical idiom can be seen in the US-developed psychiatric classification system *The Diagnostic and Statistical Manual of Mental Disorders* (DSM). This manual defines over 300 mental illnesses, most of which have been 'identified' in the last 20 years. Kutchins and Kirk (1999) suggest that the DSM has become a guidebook telling us how we should think about manifestations of sadness, anxiety, sexual activities, alcohol and substance abuse, and many other behaviours. Thus, the categories created by DSM can reorient our thinking about important social matters and affect our social institutions.

Tell me, how do you argue with a patient who has been brought in for compulsory 'treatment' when the patient argues back to you (as has happened on occasions during my years of training in adult psychiatry) saying 'I am not ill, you can take any test from me that you like, take blood, do scans, do any test you wish and show me that I am ill'. Of course, if you think about it, you realize that the patient is right. How come he is being given what is called treatment against his will, when we cannot even show any evidence that he is ill according to the norms for evidence used in the rest of medicine. Of course, this is not treatment as defined in the rest of medicine. Even if you have a life-threatening illness such as diabetes, you cannot be treated against your will. As a result psychiatry has had to put up with an allied conceptual difficulty. If compulsory treatment is not treatment as defined in the rest of medicine, is it an agent of social control (somebody has to do it)? It seems that the concepts that psychiatrists develop lend themselves well to this social political purpose.

So, what about child and adolescent psychiatry then? Is there a similar social process occurring, a process whereby psychiatrists create concepts that medicalize social and political issues, resulting in a peculiar idea of treatment on the one hand and a social, political function on behalf of the state on the other? I very much believe so. The rise and rise of the twin diagnoses of attention deficit hyperactivity disorder (ADHD) (see Chapter 7) and autism in boys reflects, I believe, the increasing failure of the education system in particular, and current western culture in general, to know how to accept, nurture and deal with boys. As the 'system' washes its hands (e.g. by expelling them from school) of having to deal with and take responsibility for ensuring the welfare of boys, so they are sent to our departments for a medical label. Then everyone can feel absolved of blame as the child has an illness. What say can children have in such a system? Their heads should be full of the adult voices from which they are learning. Instead, from early in their life we script them with an illness or disability story. Sadly for our cultural values, and happily for the pharmaceutical industry, the amount of psychotropic medication prescribed to children in the US increased nearly fourfold between 1985 and 1994 (Pincus *et al.*, 1998). The trend in modern child-psychiatric practice is for symptom-based (context deprived) assessments, use of screening question-naires, aggressive use of psychotropic medication, use of multiple prescriptions with little information about their safety or long-term consequences and a typical 15 to 20-minute medical follow-up appointment to check dosages of medication (Pincus *et al.*, 1998; Jellinek, 1999). We are in danger of becoming a skill-deprived context-starved profession.

Until psychiatry is able to develop a clear, causal framework to support its definitions, the scientific legitimacy of the definitions has to be questioned. At this present stage in psychiatry's history the belief system on which we professionals rely is a social construct of theory-driven ideas. Without a central, medical, causal basis to back the psychiatric classification systems we use, then any research using this system of classification is unlikely to yield anything of great medical significance. Thus, it is hardly surprising that all we seem to get from psychiatric research is a confused cacophony of discordant 'evidence'. For every finding on any of the major 'mental illnesses', there is another one that contradicts it. It is the same in child and adolescent psychiatry. The situation makes a mockery of evidence-based practice in this field as there is no consistent evidence, there are no proven medical bases for the problems we deal with and there are no proven treatments. The most courageous interpretation of the evidence would be to view the complete lack of consistency in the research findings as good evidence that our current classification system does not reflect any meaningful medical or naturally occurring phenomena. The evidence suggests we should dump our current psychiatric classification. It is not scientific and should stop pretending to be so.

Yet we have journal after journal producing article after article by academics who are funded to the tune of billions. The research tends to be academic, unreflective of clinical reality and rarely are the results of any research significant enough to influence clinician's practice (especially as most are aware that soon another study will come along to contradict whatever finding is being presented). The lack of a solid, scientific baseline means we are building castles on sand, the researchers carry on building without paying much attention to the fact that the sand is not a good place to start building and so the castle keeps collapsing in various places. Maybe one day it will collapse completely as more clear evidence emerges concerning the possible substrates behind mental-health difficulties. When that day arrives I am pretty sure that the existing diagnostic structure and framework will disappear completely to be replaced by a more logical one.

As there is no known pathological basis to any of the diagnoses we make (in adult and child psychiatry) and despite the strong belief that we are dealing with primarily biological disorders, most psychiatric authors are forced to conclude that the conditions we deal with have 'multifactorial' causes (are caused by many different factors). Then the fun begins, these multifactors can act together or maybe by themselves or in various combinations with different factors at play in different individuals (although we have no way of discovering or proving which factors are at play in which individuals). The 'multifactorial' conclusion looks to me like an admission of 'we don't know what the hell is going on here, so let's just throw in everything we can think of and the kitchen sink just to be sure'.

Thus, in its present state, psychiatry, including child and adolescent psychiatry, can be thought of as a culture-thick, not science-thick, social and political endeavour. Its practitioners, in their training, are being trained to use a particular cultural approach which relies on a belief system and the faith of the practitioner in that belief system, and which then imposes this belief system upon others. The discomfort of the client is particularly apparent where their belief system becomes more and more distant from that of the psychiatrist.

Psychiatry as a cultural defence mechanism

Freud once said

> There are three sources from which our suffering comes: the superior power of nature, the feebleness of our own bodies and the inadequacy of the regulations which adjust the mutual relationships of human beings in the family, the state and society . . . As regards the third source, the social source of suffering our attitude is a different one. We do not admit it at all. We cannot see why the regulations made by ourselves should not, on the contrary, be a protection and benefit for everyone of us.
>
> (Freud, 1930: 274)

This observation is right on the ball. The social source of suffering, being the most difficult to tackle, is the source of suffering that most societies do not like to admit to, and it is questionable as to whether we have made any progress in tackling it at all. With regard to the first two sources of suffering, the superior power of nature and the feebleness of our own bodies, it is very clear that the industrial revolution and accompanying scientific developments brought about very large changes in the way we are deal with these (although it is open to question whether this is progress, as modern industrial societies have a record for replacing one problem with another, e.g. global warming). Unlike these two sources of suffering which are primarily to do with physical suffering, the third source, that of social causes of suffering, is primarily to do with mental suffering. Freud suggested that all cultures struggle with this and all cultures produce ways in which this social suffering can be regulated in some manner. In fact it could be argued that culture is all about developing ways of regulating the mutual relationships of human beings in family, state and society, in other words of regulating these social causes of suffering. I believe that Freud was himself essentially proposing this reverse form/ content argument. He was in effect saying that as all cultures struggle with this question of the social causes of suffering they each produce their own sets of beliefs and values by which to regulate these most difficult areas of human life. In this light it can be seen that in the post-industrial, modernist, western societies, rationalist-inspired philosophy has provided the framework by which this culture embarked on the process of developing core belief systems by which to explain social suffering and regulate it. Just like the systems in other cultures, for example religious systems, it serves the purpose of providing a kind of social defence mechanism against the pain, discomfort, ambiguity and subjectivity of the whole complex task of trying to live as conscious human beings who are engaged in continuously trying to negotiate relationships in families, communities and societies. Extending the argument a little further, we could say that the belief systems which make up the form of the way we interpret mental-health problems are generated by and motivated by every society's need for a defence mechanism to alleviate, reduce and minimize our awareness of the mental vulnerability of the human state.

The task of raising children is one such source of 'social suffering' that tends to bring with it passionately held views. To help regulate this activity western culture has, like other cultures, developed various beliefs, values and practices that have changed over time. It is generally agreed among historians that 'modern' west European notions of childhood started taking shape in the late seventeenth century and that since then there have been a number of important shifts in the way childhood has been conceptualized (Hendrick, 1997).

In 1693 Locke published *Some Thoughts Concerning Education*, which included the idea that children were a *tabula rasa* waiting to be moulded into shape (cited in Hendrick, 1997). More significant was his idea that children were not the same, that they were individuals (Sommerville, 1982; Cunningham, 1995). In 1762 Rousseau published the highly influential *Emile*, in which he argued that children were born with innate goodness that can be corrupted by certain kinds of education (Sommerville, 1982; Hardyment, 1995). Rousseau's ideas about the 'natural child' who should be allowed to flourish soon met up with the influences of the Romantic and Evangelical revivals at the end of the eighteenth century (Hendrick, 1997).

The Romantics enveloped childhood in the concept of 'original innocence' and used this to investigate 'the self' and express the Romantic protest against the 'experience of society' (Hendrick, 1997). Then events such as the French revolution, the demand for free labour and the destruction of the old 'moral economy' pushed adult–child relations in the opposite direction to the aspirations of the Romantics. An Evangelical revival began to flourish in these new conditions and promote the idea that children are born with original sin and need redemption. The Evangelical movement had grasped the Rousseauian and Romantic ideal where childhood is portrayed as something fundamentally different to adulthood, and then used this for their own purposes (Walvin, 1982).

During the first half of the nineteenth century the debate about childhood and child rearing continued and a new construction of childhood was put together, one in which the wage-earning child was no longer to be considered the norm (Hendrick, 1997). Childhood was now seen as a separate and distinct entity requiring protection and fostering through school education. There were many influences pushing the idea of childhood and child rearing in this direction including fears about the direction of industrialization, opposition to unregulated economic activity and middle- and upper-class fears about working-class political movements. The working classes at that time were protesting against the dehumanization and brutalization of their children (Cunningham, 1995; Pearson, 1983). As the nineteenth century moved on, these ideals became incorporated into middle- and upper-class thinking. Working-class children were now seen as neglected by their parents and as a result potentially dangerous future juvenile delinquents and criminals (Pearson, 1983). It was argued that only education would prevent such 'dangerous classes' from continually reproducing malevolent characteristics and that 'parental' discipline for delinquents should be provided by reformatory schools (Pearson, 1983; May, 1973). These developments were necessary precursors to mass education and helped prepare public opinion for a further shift in the concepts of childhood and child rearing – the introduction of the state into the parent–child relationship. This happened at a time when working-class families were already having to cope with a reduction in their income. These new conditions for working-class children and their families reinforced the child's dependence and deference towards established authorities (Humphries, 1981).

Thus by the beginning of the twentieth century children were seen as individuals on whom the state could have a more fundamental influence than their families. Now that all children were in schools, they also became readily available to a variety of professionals for all sorts of 'scientific' surveys. Professional interest in the idea of child development grew and quickly became influential. Stanley Hall's writing encouraged the 'scientific' study of the individual child in order to develop an understanding of children's minds and 'guiding principles' to be offered to parents and teachers (Wooldridge, 1995). The more medically orientated Childhood Society, founded in 1897, was more interested in studying the mental and physical condition of children and especially racial considerations. Both these movements helped popularize the view that childhood is marked by stages in normal development and that there were similarities in the mental worlds of children and so-called 'primitives' (Wooldridge, 1995).

In the first half of the twentieth century a greater emphasis was placed on the involvement of children in a consciously designed pursuit of national interest, which included promoting education, racial hygiene, responsible parenthood, social purity and preventative medicine (Hendrick, 1994). In each of these areas the state was becoming more interventionist through legislation. Both state and charitable welfare organizations made a number of assumptions (many derived from psychomedicine) about what constituted 'normal' childhood. There was now a concern with 'children's' rights and an assumption that only the state could enforce these rights (Cunningham, 1995; Hendrick, 1997, 1994). These developments in childhood ideology had the effect of 'universalizing' children's development and needs and consolidated the idea of childhood as a period marked by vulnerability and requiring the protection of the state.

The inter-war period saw further refinements in the psychological conceptualization of childhood, through various strands of psychology, psychiatry, psychoanalysis and the growth of the Child Guidance Clinic movement (Wooldridge, 1995). Children were now talked about as having inner worlds of unconscious wishes, fantasies and fears, whose significance reached into adulthood and touched all our lives. Guiding children through these turbulent unconscious developmental conflicts was felt to be of great importance, not only for adult happiness, but for efficient functioning of the family and ultimately for political stability (Riley, 1983). Mothers were now told that for optimum mental development, children should be free to choose their own form of expression (Rose, 1985).

Through the development of Child Guidance Clinics in the 1920s and 1930s, child psychiatry was first consolidated as a distinct discipline within medicine. These clinics came to be viewed as a vital part of a comprehensive welfare programme. Furthermore, these clinics became important propagandists in promoting certain views about tolerant, sympathetic parenting, through radio talks, popular publications, lectures and through its association with parent–teacher organizations (Rose, 1985).

The Second World War brought with it the mass evacuation of nearly a million children, in the UK, from large industrial cities to rural reception areas. Subsequent studies of these children and their experiences contributed towards the development of psychological theories that emphasized the importance of family relationships. John Bowlby was particularly influential in developing theories about the biological nature of children's attachment to their main caregiver (1969, 1973). Separation from the main caregiver, it was suggested, was the root cause of antisocial behaviour (Rose, 1990). The 1940s also brought the 'welfare state' into being in the UK. Citizens now had the right to free social and health services. This deliberate democratization of citizenship was partly in response to post-war reconstruction and its optimistic promises, and it was partly to combat the growth of communism in Europe and nationalism in the Empire (Hendrick, 1997). Acts of parliament gave local authorities powers to become responsible for a child's care, with the idea that the publicly cared for child was to be treated as an individual with rights and possessions (Hendrick, 1994).

So we come into contemporary western society with children viewed as individuals who have rights and a need to express their opinions. They are also viewed as potentially vulnerable requiring a family (particularly a 'good-enough' mother) for optimal development and needing protection by the state when parents are deemed not to be adequate. The role of the state in intervening in family life was further increased through the 'discovery' of sexual abuse in the 1980s and the greater awareness of physical abuse. Children's rights movements gained momentum. This has been reflected in legal developments in the UK, for example the 1985 Gillick judgement where the legality of doctors giving contraceptive advice to children without parental knowledge or consent was upheld and the abolition in 1986 of corporal punishment in state schools.

At the same time as a growth in the children's rights movement, there has been a growing debate and belief that childhood in modern western society has suffered a strange death (Jenhs, 1996). Many contemporary observers voice concern about the increase in violence and disturbance amongst a generation who are perceived to have been given the best of everything (Seabrook, 1982). There is also concern about the so-called end of the innocence of childhood, for example through the greater sexualization and commercialization of childhood interests (Humphries *et al.*, 1988). The most powerful and controversial thesis has been advanced by the American sociologist, Neil Postman (1983), who claims that because of media such as television childhood is disappearing. He claims that the child has near complete access to the world of adult information which is further encouraged through things such as child models, development of children's clothes to resemble adult fashion and the replacement of traditional street games by organized junior sports leagues. In this climate, it is claimed, there has been a collapse of adult authority (Cunningham, 1995). Coupled with this fear that the boundary between childhood and adulthood is disappearing is a growing sense that children themselves are the risk, with some children being viewed as too dangerous for society, while others must be controlled, reshaped and changed (Stephens, 1995).

As social, cultural and political circumstances in modern western culture have changed, so have the attitudes to children and child rearing. Our visions of what we want our children to be and how to achieve this alters with the changing discourse. In the context of modern capitalist market economies children and their 'needs' have come to be viewed as legitimate targets for expansion of consumer markets. There is widespread concern about the breakdown of authority over children at the same time as children are being portrayed as individuals who need to express themselves, are vulnerable to abuse and need state protection. These are ideal cultural preconditions for the growth of a medical view that many of these vulnerable or out of control children cannot help they way they behave as they are ill. Thus, instead of reasserting adult authority and risking allegations of 'abuse', we can 'treat' their medical condition. This process is, of course, actively encouraged by the pharmaceutical industry as it sees another market opening up. The expansion of medical child psychiatry and the explosion in the numbers and amounts of psychoactive drugs being prescribed to children are thus part of modern western culture's attempt to regulate this area of social relationship. It is intimately tied up with current social defence mechanisms. This is one of the ways we regulate this area of potential social suffering.

The concern is that this particular social defence mechanism, despite its hierarchical position, contributes to an unhelpful avoidance of issues and the active repression of certain vulnerable groups. It is in my opinion that child and adolescent psychiatry in its present form is too disengaged from looking at and understanding its broader political and social function and therefore, all too often, is contributing to a silencing of other potentially more important voices. As culture and history moves on, child and adolescent psychiatry is in danger of being left behind, adhering to forms of practice that lack the flexibility and creativity that is needed for post-modern multicultural societies.

Chapter 5

Mental-health power hierarchies

When a cultural gap exists between two parties who is responsible for its reduction?

Do those in a position of power seek to reduce this gap or do they use their position of power to impose their model and belittle that of the other party? This latter process is that of colonization.

If you followed my argument in the last two chapters you will have realized that I believe that the whole mental-health business is about belief systems rather than hard science. Still, we all need belief systems to regulate our lives and to give some social and cultural structure to our continuing attempts to regulate the suffering that comes about through being human and through being in human relationships. I am also suggesting that when you look at it from this point of view all cultures are doing the same thing. As far as the ultimate validity or truth of any of these systems, on the whole all are fallible, a fact that psychiatry has to acknowledge if it is to make genuine scientific progress.

In this chapter I want to concentrate on the issue of power hierarchies as it is these power dynamics that dictate which belief systems become dominant, which ones are belittled and how this then translates into the clinical practice of mental-health professionals working with children, adolescents and families. These power hierarchies also influence culture in general and our cultural beliefs about what is desirable, acceptable and normal for children, adolescents, family life, future aspirations, dependency, child rearing, discipline and so on. With so much pathologizing and blame around, it is hard constantly struggling against a cultural discourse that makes you feel small, a failure, unvalued and a waste of space.

Discourse and power

In our everyday lives we are all surrounded by conversations, stories, articles, interviews, programmes, books, newspapers, television, radio, friends, relatives and colleagues who are all in the process of passing or exchanging information with us. The stories we hear, conversations we have, articles we read and programmes we watch all contribute to our understanding of the world around us. We filter the stories and interpret them according to our belief systems, we take up some and challenge others, we interpret the same story differently, and so on. These constant social events around us are the way that culture informs our thinking and beliefs. This starts from a very young age and carries on throughout our lives. As our beliefs develop we use them as a framework and a reference point by which to interpret the stories that we hear, the world around us and the problems in living that we encounter.

Naturally, the stories that you hear and the beliefs that you develop vary from individual to individual, family to family, community to community, nation to nation and culture to culture. The stories I heard and the beliefs I was surrounded by when growing up in Iraq were very different compared to the beliefs, lifestyle and attitudes I encountered when I came to England. In school in Iraq, I was taught in classes with rows of desks, a blackboard at the front and a teacher with a thick ruler in her hand to police classroom behaviour and who was not afraid to use this ruler at the slightest infringement of the rules. There were standard textbooks for the whole country and we would often recite after the teacher to learn by rote many things. I lived in an extended family environment, always surrounded by lots of people, cousins, aunts, uncles and friends, coming and going, listening to their stories about religion and God. There were outings with lots of families to date plantations south of Basra, to fir-tree forests on the edge of the desert. There was dirt and the stench of sewage in the summer, the call to prayer ringing out over the city five times a day and a queue of people waiting to affectionately pinch my cheeks. Children were loved and it was obvious. Then when I was 14 years old we had to come to England. I found myself in colourful classrooms with children who thought nothing of joking with a teacher or answering them back. Suddenly, not to be overtly sexually interested in girls meant you were a 'poof' (the opposite of what I'd just left behind, where at this age boys were not expected to show interest in girls). Self-esteem, learning self-control and individuality were more obvious (what was this self-esteem thing? what did it mean?). Families lived in a private space. Food and material goods poured out of shop windows. Wow, freedom. In the papers I read today I can sense the ambivalence about children – they are either demonized as evil killers, drug abusers, bullies and muggers, or romanticized as victims of abuse and trauma from day one in their lives. Children just seem to get in the way. When I go out with my own children now I am on constant alert to complaining voices, your children are too loud, badly behaved, brats. Few seem to break into a smile of genuine pleasure at the innocence and wonder of the growing child.

When you come into training as a mental-health professional you enter an environment which has particular stories to tell, beliefs to pass on and methods to instill. It stands to reason that this professional culture and the types of stories, ideas, articles, books, and discussions that you are going to be surrounded by will have a significant impact on your professional beliefs about health and ill health, how to identify it, and how to deal with it. For all psychiatrists this process begins during the medical-school training. Conventional medical training teaches students to view medicine as a science with the clinician as an impartial investigator who builds differential diagnoses as if they were scientific theories excluding competing possibilities, in a manner that is similar to disproving a hypothesis. There is an assumption which is present from very early on in the professional training that clinical observation and data collection is an objective exercise and, like all scientific measurements, reproducible. While some of this core attitude may hold true in branches of medicine where objective material facts on individual patients are obtainable (although even in much of the rest of medicine there are many grey areas which are theory driven), in psychiatry there really are no objective material facts to back up any of the theories that you apply to any individual patient. Diagnoses in psychiatry are derived from a purely theory-driven account of observable behaviour and information elicited from the patient and informants.

So when the psychiatrist carries this ideology into the mental-health arena, they already have a set of internalized beliefs and, more importantly, a practice methodology that has been highly influenced by the dominant medical model. The child psychiatrist will have then undergone a training in general adult psychiatry before entering the 'sub-specialty' of child and adolescent psychiatry. The years of general psychiatry will no doubt have further exposed the child psychiatrist-to-be to the dominant medical model approach, as well as to the hierarchical nature of service organization. In modern mental-health services, the psychiatrist remains the ultimate decision maker. In the current systems, mental health is an issue and responsibility primarily for doctors who are believed to hold the most advanced knowledge and expertise in relation to these problems of living.

All being well in this system, the child and adolescent psychiatrist should arrive into their chosen specialty believing that they can claim a legitimate position at the head of the table, as they bring the highest level of scientific knowledge by which to evaluate and treat childhood mental-health disorders. All being well they will have brought the supremacy of the medical model with them. Of course, during their training they will have been exposed to some elements from competing frameworks for understanding the mental-health problems of children. Some may even have completed some formal training in one of these fields (e.g. child psychotherapy, family therapy). But too much non-medical influence makes the profession feel jittery. The child-psychiatry professor who was the organizer of the academic part of my child-psychiatry training, always claimed that we were doomed to a terrible decline if we didn't become more like real doctors (presumably with stethoscope and prescription pad in hand). Thus in child and adolescent psychiatry in the UK today, there is a powerful lobby arguing that we need to become more 'doctory'. I firmly believe that this is pushing our profession backwards towards a pseudo-doctor role, despite the complete lack of any objective factual medical tests to back up the claims for a medical basis to the conditions that child and adolescent psychiatrists spend their time diagnosing. Some claim that this is a way of decreasing the medicalization of children's problems (e.g. Goodman, 1997). This is the opposite of what an approach such as this actually does. Rates of diagnosis for conditions such as attention deficit hyperactivity disorder (ADHD) and autism have rocketed in the last 10 years, as have the rates and amounts of psychotropic medication being given to children and adolescents (see Chapters 4 and 7). Anybody working in a child and adolescent psychiatry department or a community paediatric department will tell you that. Why? Because these conditions cannot be medically defined they end up being hugely influenced by social trends with a kind of elastic-band effect, whereby the boundaries of the disorder stretch to accommodate an ever-widening easy way out for practitioners to not think about complex problems (and beliefs about what constitutes a problem). This is a grave mistake. It results in a rigid, tunnel-vision view whereby children and their problems are stripped of any context. It's a kind of original-sin model that pathologizes children (particularly boys) in ever increasing numbers. Children's psyche is being carved up as if it was an entity separated from its environment, an entity that the psychiatrist understands. I have seen reports written by child psychiatrists in which they state 'he has a condition in which 80 per cent of his behaviour is hereditary and thus beyond his control'. How the hell did the psychiatrist work that one out? We must curb this ridiculous pseudo-medicine. Psychiatry should not be a branch of surgery carving up people's psyche and dismembering them from their reality.

Frameworks in child and adolescent mental health are competing for the same ground and trying to define the same territory. So why do some frameworks come out as having greater status and an overarching superiority by which services are organized, research is driven, journalists are informed, articles and programmes are made, and the general cultural climate of a community and country's approach to childhood and its problems are influenced? Power hierarchies have a lot to do with this.

There are many manifestations of power, the most obvious being coercion. There are also many other ways in which influence and power is wielded. These more subtle and insidious ways of maintaining a powerful position can be more difficult to deal with as they are often unseen and therefore more difficult emotionally to challenge. This is particularly so if they are accompanied by attempts to disguise the intentions of those wishing to hold on to their positions of power. Other than coercion, power can be wielded in ways that include the suppression of conflicts and differences, and owning the means to produce consensus by holding positions that allow you to have a major influence on local discourse (Luke, 1974; Weingarten, 1998).

Such power dynamics affecting the dominant discourse lead to frameworks for understanding life's problems, and for establishing a social pecking order for the relative status and importance each framework is afforded and the cultural profile it is given. There is little doubt that in the current western (so-called modernist era), psychiatrists have the highest status as spokespeople for understanding the mental health of children and adolescents, and as the dominant framework used to organize thinking, service delivery and research. The power of the psychiatric framework is such that in our culture, and in most cultures around the world, everybody is familiar with the idea of mental illness; with illness being defined and thought about in the same way that we think about illness in the rest of medicine, that is as having something physically wrong with you. Coming close behind illness is the label 'disorder'. By using words like 'illness' and 'disorder', psychiatrists are manipulating language to convey the impression of something medical or physical being wrong which therefore can only be understood and treated by a doctor.

With the medical model having such high status and extending its tentacles ever wider into children's lives and their problems, deficit models overwhelm us. The great pathologizers of childhood spend time and energy convincing us that there is more ADHD, autism, childhood depression, obsessive compulsive disorder, eating disorders and so on, than we are recognizing and treating. They call for more training into how to recognize these disorders, so we can all join the pathologizing schools of thought. Perhaps we want perfect children (an ever receding will-o-the wisp). Perhaps there are real increases in these disorders, in which case what is the environmental cause(s) for this? Perhaps we're just good at getting ourselves more and more jobs (child and adolescent psychiatry is an expanding specialty). Whatever the reason, it remains that it is the psychiatrist who is given ultimate status for defining the cultural common sense on what constitutes a mental-health problem for children and adolescents.

To better understand how psychiatry has achieved such status and continues to occupy this high status some historical context is useful.

A brief history of psychiatry

The history of psychiatry is a peculiar and contradictory one. Whilst the rest of medicine has a history punctuated by dramatic and decisive breakthroughs in understanding the nature and aetiology of disease, mental medicine can claim few such successes. This major difference is reflected in the types of historical accounts available of the history of psychiatry. If we inspect historical accounts of, say, the development of modern biology or chemistry, or within medical history of, say, surgery or anaesthetics, we find essential agreement on subject matters, developmental themes and transformational episodes, that are central and constitutive of the discipline. The same cannot be claimed for the history of psychiatry. Modern psychiatry has come about, not through the steady unproblematic accumulation of ideas and practices through the centuries, but sporadically, with periods of little advance, stagnation and some would say regression. Both empirically and interpretively, the histories of psychiatry reveal a vast degree of difference among themselves than historical accounts of any other discipline.

Psychiatry has always been fighting off other professions and disciplines interested in the same field of enquiry, to try and maintain medical supremacy. Mythology, hypnotism, theology, philosophy, law, anthropology, literature, lay healing, sociology, psychology, the therapies, complimentary and other older forms of medicine, spiritual healing and so on have all laid claim at one time or another to certain aspects of the mental-health arena. Furthermore, the subject matter of psychiatry has continually shifted. Poised precariously between the medical sciences and the human sciences, mental medicine has routinely lost, then gained, then lost again its disciplinary territory as neighbouring fields expand and contract (Rosenberg, 1975). With an intensely subjective subject matter, an insecure and shifting epistemological base, porous interdisciplinary boundaries and a sectarian and dialectical dynamic of development, it has thus proved impossible to produce anything like an enduring and comprehensive history of psychiatry (Hunter and Macalpine, 1963). Instead rather opposing styles, reflecting on the history of psychiatry, exist.

One style is that of the uncritical 'in-house' historical accounts, written by psychiatrists, about psychiatrists and for psychiatrists, which tend to be self-congratulatory in nature. For example

> After the tortures and judicial murders of the middle ages and the renaissance, which confounded demonical possession with delusion and frenzy, and smelt out witchcraft in the maunderings of demented old women, there were the cruelties and degradation of the madhouses of the seventeenth and eighteenth centuries . . . In the nineteenth century, the pathology of insanity was investigated, its clinical forms described and classified its kinship with physical disease and psychoneurosis recognised. Treatment was undertaken in university hospitals and out patient clinics multiplied . . . In the twentieth century, psychopathology has been elucidated and psychological treatment given ever widening scope and sanction. Revolutionary changes have occurred in physical methods of treatment; the regime in mental hospitals has been further liberalised.
>
> (Lewis, 1967: 3)

This uncritical self aggrandizement of psychiatry by psychiatrists continues to this day.

> There is a broad consensus within psychiatry, a consensus that has strengthened in recent years, to the effect that the advantages of the disease approach, the diagnostic process and the present rudimentary classification system, outweigh the disadvantages.
>
> (Clare, 1997: 52)

At the beginning of the 1960s a cluster of authors, in re-interpreting the status of progress in psychiatry, provoked the beginning of a great revision in the understanding of psychiatric history. Goffman's *Asylums* (1961), Laing's *The Divided Self* (1960), Szasz's *The Myth of Mental Illness* (1961) and Foucault's *Historie de la Folie* (1961), all questioned the official assurances of the fundamental benignity of the psychiatric enterprise, as well as its claims to be a scientific medical discipline that we need more of.

In the 1970s, a mixture of disaffected psychotherapists, radical sociologists and academic historians produced more historical accounts that questioned the central claim of psychiatry to be a medical discipline offering medical treatment, stressing instead the covert social and moral normalizing political function of the discipline.

Amongst these, Doerner's *Burger und Irre* (1969) Rothman's *The Discovery of the Asylum* (1971), Castel's *L'Ordre Psychiatrique* (1976) and Scull's *Museums of Madness* (1979), were to prove influential.

The re-authoring and re-interpreting of psychiatric history paints the discipline as one that has essentially failed in its stated aims and that continues to occupy its hierarchical status for social, political and cultural reasons and most certainly not for its record of success.

Psychiatrists, however, have been good at fighting their corner, presumably aided by the growing status and record of success of other spheres of medicine. When, in the nineteenth century a lay person, William Tuke, and his colleagues began to claim success for their 'moral treatment' in the asylum they ran in York, doctors acted to make sure their claims to have special skills to treat the insane was not threatened: 'The disease of insanity in all its shades and varieties belongs, in point of treatment, to the department of the physician alone . . . the medical treatment is that part on which the whole success of the cure lies' (Hill, quoted in Scull, 1979: 135). Doctors argued successfully against legislation that would mean that a growing number of public asylums would come under the supervision and control of a board of lay people. Doctors insisted that only medical experts could undertake this task satisfactorily, consolidating their victory with a spate of medical articles, lists of diagnosis, and lectures on the treatment of insanity becoming a part of normal medical training. Of course, this still left doctors with the problem of demonstrating the physical basis for the conditions they were now claiming sole expertise over. On the promise that proof would be forthcoming in time, doctors experimented with all manner of physical treatments. The remedies tried included injections of morphia, administration of bromides, chloral hydrate, hypocymine, cannabis, amyl nitrate, conium, digitalis, ergot, pilocarpine, emetics, purgatives, sudden immersion in cold water, pouring 10 to 50 buckets of icy water on patients' heads, raising blisters on the head and neck and rubbing salves into the pustules, applying leeches or ants to the skin, whipping with stinging nettles, making incisions on the skin, applying red-hot pokers simultaneously to the head and the soles of the feet, drilling holes in the scalp, putting patients in revolving chairs, applying restraining masks to the face, being bathed in gruel, milk or gravy, and putting patients on the treadmill for long periods (Kraepelin, 1962).

Over the last 100 years, the medical profession has continued to consolidate its monopoly over the treatment of the mentally distressed. Physical treatments such as insulin-coma therapy, electric-shock treatment and psychosurgery were to become popular in the early twentieth century. Psychiatry then showed its potential for use as a political agent for the state, in the ultimate show of its social control credentials by becoming involved in the eugenics movement in Nazi Germany. The psychiatric profession actively collaborated first with the compulsory sterilization of about 400,000 people said to be suffering from hereditary mental illnesses or learning disabilities, and then in the mass killing of about 100,000 German psychiatric patients, mostly in gas chambers strategically located close to psychiatric clinics across the country (Meyer, 1998; Burleigh, 1994).

In the 1950s and 1960s new classes of medication, namely the major tranquillizers (or anti-psychotics), the anti-depressants, lithium and the minor tranquillizers (or benzodiazepines) brought new claims of miracle cures. The alternative historical account and interpretation suggests otherwise. There are some interesting parallels between the nineteenth century issues and debates and the present-day ones. Then as now psychiatry was devoting itself to proving that mental distress has a physical origin. Now as then, despite the continuing lack of physical and empirical evidence, the reliance on physical treatments to back psychiatrists' claims and maintain their hegemony continues. Now as then explanations of how these treatments are meant to work are speculative. Now as then the number of cures that physical treatments are providing remains distressingly low. Now as then there is no shortage of jargon and lists of diagnoses to give the whole field an air of expertise and authority. Modern psychiatry, like that of a century ago, makes great claims for the success of medical treatments. These claims have thus far either proved inaccurate (e.g. that major tranquillizers enable chronic patients to be discharged from hospitals for good) or consisted of belated recognition of the potential harmfulness of some of its treatments (e.g. the addictive effects of minor tranquillizers) (Johnstone, 2000).

A brief history of child psychiatry

Child and adolescent psychiatry has grown out of a similar mixture of inter-disciplinary rivalry and competing professional interests. As in general psychiatry, doctors have used their status and social or political privilege to assert themselves to the top of this field, with the result that more and more children's problems are being conceptualized within a medical framework.

With child psychiatry being a relatively young profession, having only begun to separate from general psychiatry a little over 50 to 80 years ago (Black, 1993), there are few outside the profession who have analysed the history of child psychiatry from a critical viewpoint. All that is readily available at present is the self-congratulatory historical accounts by child psychiatrists for child psychiatrists. Child psychiatry first established itself as a separate medical discipline within the influential, psychoanalytically orientated Child Guidance Clinic movement of the 1920s and 1930s (see Chapter 4). The Child Guidance Clinic movement had an important impact on cultural attitudes to children and child rearing, encouraging tolerant, sympathetic parenting, an emphasis on the importance of the mother–child relationship and on talking to your children (Hendrick, 1997). As the profession gained momentum in the latter half of the twentieth century, the inevitable claims about the commonness of childhood psychiatric disorder (affecting 7 to 20 per cent of children according to Rutter et al., 1970a, 1970b) and its massive under-recognition (less than 1 per cent of children being seen in child-psychiatry departments according to Kolvin, 1973) came. Over the last 20 to 30 years of the twentieth century the profession built up its power base, took over the running of Child Guidance Clinics and presided over their demise. In their place academic departments and Child and Adolescent Mental Health Service clinics were set up.

Child psychiatrists firmed up their position as the highest-paid consultants in child and adolescent mental-health services. Leading child psychiatrists were pleased that after some difficult turbulent years before establishing itself at the top of the hierarchy, child psychiatry could now claim to have developed a firm scientific basis and an evidence-based expertise that together with good leadership skills had put the profession in a healthy position (Graham, 1976; Rutter, 1986).

The alternative history would show a similar story to that in adult psychiatry, of a profession whose dominance owes more to cultural fashion and politics than to any notable medical advance. More and more child psychiatry has to do with the social project of 'normalizing' misfit children, particularly those who do not fit well into the current education system. It is no surprise to me that boys do not achieve at school as well as girls these days and that at the same time we seem to be having an epidemic of the fashionable boy diagnosis, ADHD (see Chapter 7).

Cultural influences on psychiatric thinking

Of course, mental-health theories have not grown up in a cultural vacuum. As well as influencing and informing everyday culture, everyday culture has influenced and informed mental-health ideologies. Therefore it is hardly surprising to see how, historically, the dominant theories have been driven by notions of the ideal or healthy state, being defined by the dominant discourses of the time. Retrospectively, we can also recognize that prevailing cultural ideology has been challenged and changed by mental-health theories too. For example, Freud challenged the whole notion of sexuality and many of the prevailing cultural beliefs about the instincts. His ideas were to have a massive and continuing impact on beliefs about a whole range of issues from child rearing to art critique.

It is also possible to see cultural shifts in a number of areas, which have then affected mental-health theory and definitions. For example, psychoanalysis has been criticized for paying too much attention to fantasy and not enough to reality and therefore minimizing the issue of sexual abuse. Following a shift in cultural attitudes in the 1970s and 1980s, childhood sexual abuse became more widely acknowledged as a real (as opposed to fantasized) traumatic event. Homosexuality used to be classified as a psychiatric disorder being seen as an illness, until its removal from psychiatric categories occurred when cultural attitudes shifted in the latter half of the last century.

White, male, middle-class, doctors and other academics have been the predominant force in constructing psychiatric, and its younger sibling child and adolescent psychiatric, notions. It is therefore hardly surprising to find that psychiatric and psychological theory tends to produce clinical practice that defines pathology, ill health and dysfunction in a way that replicates the dominant cultural beliefs of this group. This has resulted in a classification system that either describes pathology, or is interpreted by the practitioner, in a way that can marginalize the experience of many socially disadvantaged groups along the lines of race, culture, class, gender and sexuality. There are no discussions of the power relationships and there is a complete lack of insight into the influence that these issues may have in shaping, not only mental-health theories and our professional beliefs and practices, but also the mental experiences of our clients and the wider cultural group.

The way in which we professionals negatively define people, their lives and their life problems is, inevitably, dominated by cultural attitudes derived from our own cultural background in general and our professional cultural background in particular. The definitions we create leave us in a position of power to impose these negative mental-health theories and practices on those who are less powerful (see Chapter 3). It is not surprising therefore to find constant over-representation of different disadvantaged social groups in most psychiatric categories. This pattern shows in child-psychiatric practice, as its diagnoses become more fashionable (e.g. the over-representation of children from a working-class background in the diagnosis of ADHD, see Chapter 7).

In developing our professional ideas about what constitutes normal childhood and child-rearing practice, we inevitably draw on the concepts that have been developed in western culture (see Chapter 4 for a discussion on how childhood has come to be conceptualized in the west). Our professional notions of a deviant childhood, while acknowledging differences in children's lives, has also legitimized universal notions of the ideal childhood (Stephens, 1995). And it is not only citizens of the developed west whom it is believed should have our particular sort of child-hood, but also populations around the world who are seen as in need of 'civilization' and 'development'. In the past 20 to 30 years there has been increasing media coverage of developing countries' children, whose lives appear strikingly different to the idealized western childhood (James and Prout, 1990). These 'deviant child-hoods' of children from developing countries are often considered to be backward, and this has justified the export of modern western notions of childhood around the world. All too often the media representation of the conditions of material poverty that many children from developing countries live in (that has, arguably, been caused by western capitalism), is equated with inner poverty.

The export of the politically powerful western cultural notions of childhood to the less powerful nations can be illustrated by examining how the debate on children's rights was developed in the United Nations. The foundation for a global standard for children's rights was laid down in 1959, when the UN General Assembly adopted the Declaration of the Rights of the Child. The Declaration specified a series of rights for children that were largely phrased in terms of general moral entitlements, for example the 'right to love and understand'. The Declaration was aimed at protecting and nurturing childhood, as defined by adults within the framework of western modernity. It did not recognize that there might be cultural differences in what constitutes children's best interests (Boyden, 1990). In 1989 the UN General Assembly adopted the UN Convention on the Rights of the Child. Unlike the 1959 Declaration, the 1989 Convention is not just a general statement of good intent, but is considered legally binding for ratifying states.

One of the qualitatively new aspects of the Convention is an emphasis on the capacity of the child to act, at least partially, independently of adults. Thus the convention lays down rights, such as the child's right to freedom of expression, that are not just protective (Cantwell, 1989). It seems that in the name of universal rights for children, what actually happened was one dominant cultural historical framework for understanding childhood was asserted in a way that made other cultures subordinate. Indeed the majority of the countries from the south voiced criticisms of the predominantly western notions of normal childhood and child rearing underlying the Convention (Fyfe, 1989). Even the language of the Convention talks about the rights of the 'child' as opposed to children, thus emphasizing the individualized freestanding child. The preamble describes the family as 'the fundamental group of society and the natural environment for the growth and well-being of its members' (Stephens, 1995: 37). This description implies that the western nuclear family should be the norm, making other family forms such as extended, multigenerational, single parent and so on appear deviant (Stephens, 1995). The child's right to education is developed with a view to eliminating 'ignorance and illiteracy throughout the world and facilitating access to scientific and technical knowledge and modern teaching methods' (Stephens, 1995: 37). This calls into question the importance of local religious teaching and orally transmitted values (Stephens, 1995). The question of identity is treated as an individual right (i.e. identity is individualized) with culture not even mentioned as a central element for most children's identity. The convention even goes on to state that countries must take effective measures to abolish traditional practices prejudicial to the health of children, presumably from a western biomedical perspective. Boyden (1990) concludes that the UN, as a mediator of liberal democratic rule globally, has been vested with a strong interest in spreading to poor countries of the south, the values and practices of the industrialized north.

In many ways it seems that modern western capitalism has done to childhood what it continues to do to the poor countries of the world. First the space of childhood was colonized (and the boundary between adults and children melted, opening up tremendously lucrative markets). The guilty conscience that this produced helped spurn a children's rights movement. This in turn could be exploited to increase the state's control over children and thus give back childhood its space but in the way that western authorities would like it to be (so as not to conflict with economic interests). Now this vision is being exported in the same old colonial way. We will take away and colonize your values and practices and when you protest we will give you back the right to remake yourselves in our own image.

Modern child psychiatry is a full participant in this process. A culturally western image of the ideal childhood and child-rearing methods is the foundation for defining psychiatric deviance. These definitions are imposed on all communities and exported worldwide. Thus Hodes (1998) decides refugee children require a lot of psychiatric help. He concludes that about half of the population of refugee children have a 'serious' psychiatric disorder that requires western-inspired psychological and psychiatric treatments. Glaser (1993) describes what she believes emotional abuse of children to be. She includes such things as belittlement, refusing to speak to the child, exposure to feared stimuli, making continued care conditional upon the child's behaviour or gratitude, induction of guilt or terror to promote compliance, inappropriate expectations or imposed responsibilities, using the child to obtain vicarious satisfaction for the parent and involvement of the child in coercively applied ideological systems, in her list of what constitutes emotionally abusive behaviour by a parent. The highly subjective middle-class western nature of her thinking is revealed more clearly by the categories she uses to describe practices such as the above. Her four categories of emotional abuse are persistent negative attitudes, use of guilt and fear as the predominant disciplinary practices, ignorance or exploitation of the child's immature developmental status and distorted recognition of the child's individuality. Her vision of childhood emotional abuse is built on modern western notions of the importance of individuality, freedom of expression and the Children's Rights Movement's emphasis on childhood as a period marked by special vulnerability. I attended one of Dr Glaser's seminars during my training and asked her how these definitions for emotional abuse translate cross-culturally. She told me that it means that maybe 80 per cent to 90 per cent of children from developing countries could be categorized as having been abused.

Hierarchy and power in daily clinical contexts

Within the psychiatric profession straightforward coercion is rife. During my years of training as a junior-grade psychiatrist and then child psychiatrist, I have been forced to prescribe drugs at toxic doses, send adults and children to secure units and sometimes have been silenced from voicing any concerns by threats such as 'you'll get a reputation and then no one will employ you', 'it's clear to me you don't understand medical hierarchy, until you do you should not be working here', 'I know a lot of consultants nationally and I could make it very difficult for you to get a job as a consultant', 'we need to look at whether you are suited to working in this profession', to recall but a few. It has been confusing, as many consultants I've worked for have been very complimentary about my work. Some, it seems, can't deal with any challenges to their way of thinking and are prone to use their position to bully you into compliance. As a consultant too, I have also unfortunately had to work with other consultants who are prone to flexing their muscles to try and get you to fall into line with their version of psychiatry, despite our equal status. When I volunteered to set up a local ADHD clinic (see Chapter 7), the clinic committee chaired by the clinic lead (another consultant) initially rejected it. I was told that my proposal (which had the complete backing of colleagues and parents involved in developing the proposal in the first place) did not look like an ADHD clinic as it was clearly not the expert led (i.e. medical-model-dominated) clinic they had wanted to establish. I then had to go through the process of resigning from being the lead for establishing this clinic (stating that if they already knew what sort of clinic they wanted then somebody else should take the lead for establishing this clinic), suffering a complaint being made about me by the clinic lead, meetings with management, and re-jargonizing the proposal in a way that would give it superficial acceptance by the clinic committee, before finally being able to get on with developing and running the clinic as we had intended.

Marginalization, divide and rule, a them-and-us mentality is another way of maintaining power. In consultants' meetings, some cannot seem to stop talking about power, threats to power, and the necessity for psychiatrists to maintain power and the belittling of other professional groups' capabilities. If you don't agree with this dogma, then you get subtle messages that you are no longer one of us. You find yourself not consulted about certain decisions, not invited to certain meetings, and not expected to be part of certain management groups. Sometimes this can result in an atmosphere of paranoia and suspicion. You start to read between the lines, you feel you are not valued, you feel your work might be criticized or worse seen as 'off the wall'. If this gets bad you isolate yourself in a protective self-fulfilling prophecy, living your professional life on the margins of the institution. Alternatively you can become the 'madman' who will be dismissed as having a chip on their shoulder, an 'off they go again' sort of thing as soon as you open your mouth. If it's really bad you'll do both and feel yourself going crazy. I've been through this and seen others go through this. Challenging the mainstream can be a lonely, isolating experience. I have wondered if this is what it's like for many of the clients I see daily surviving social exclusion and marginalization as they fight to keep sane, to stop feeling so small, powerless and manipulated. Perhaps this is the experience Fanon (1967) was talking about when he said that black families in Europe often had to choose between alienation or adopting a European outlook and pretending that the racism around them did not exist.

Alongside marginalization as a tactic, go conflict suppression, denial and avoidance. Conflicts can be glossed over as a way of avoiding looking at differences of opinion. The whole general psychiatric and child-psychiatric training makes absolutely no mention and gives no voice to anti-psychiatry, critical psychiatry or user organizations. The debate about the basic disagreements that exist over the fundamental concepts, on which psychiatry is based, is simply treated as if it did not exist. I've had a consultant whom I worked alongside, who knew I had an Arabic father and had grown up in an Arabic country, tell me she hates visiting Arabic countries because of 'the way they treat their women'. I believe she genuinely did not consider or realize that this had offended me, as she probably assumed that by now I identified with the majority professional view that men from developing countries (compared to western men) treat women badly.

Power hierarchies manifest themselves constantly in clinical situations. If your ideas, beliefs and values are from a cultural system with low status and low acceptance, then would you let those high-status clinicians know about them? Would they laugh at you? Would they try and patronize you by being sympathetic, yet try to convince you that your ideas are ignorant, superstitious and foolish? Would they try to educate you about mental illness, psychiatric disorder and good parenting? If you become defensive would they look down their noses at you? Would you become paranoid and start reading between the lines? Is that really what they mean when they say 'yes, I understand what you're saying'? I've seen

13 riot police arrive on a ward I worked on to help with the forcible injection of tranquillizing medication into a newly admitted, young black man with no previous known psychiatric history because he was said to be 'staring in a threatening manner'. I've seen a 13-year-old Asian girl medicated and admitted to a secure unit against her and her parents' wishes because the consultant believed she was dangerously psychotic, when her problems were no more than temper outbursts. I've seen bucket loads of reports on post-overdose adolescent girls from Asian families that talk about how repressive the parents are and the importance of persuading the families to allow more western-style freedom. I've listened to truck loads of clinicians knee jerking their way to labelling working-class parents as incompetent and abusive.

Of course things can proceed smoothly. If the client comes to the professional with the belief that they may have a particular mental illness for which medication could be helpful, and they share a similar cultural and social background with the clinician who then sets about establishing a diagnosis and suggesting a drug treatment, then it is easy to see that such an interview may proceed smoothly with both parties feeling satisfied about the outcome. However, the greater the differences between the clinician's and the client's belief systems the greater the discomfort. This is particularly so for the clinician, who will have a great temptation to impose his/her belief system and belittle that of the client, a process which I believe can have adverse consequences on clients already struggling with feelings of difference, inferiority and the distress this brings.

The hierarchy by which services are organized is deeply embedded both in the service culture and in the wider culture generally. Other professionals often feel forced to refer up to psychiatrists even though they are usually perfectly capable of dealing with their clients themselves. Many clients request to be seen by a psychiatrist, with the belief that seeing the psychiatrist means getting access to the most knowledgeable 'expert'. Many agencies (social services, education) specifically request psychiatric assessments, with phrases such as 'in order to discover what is wrong with him', 'to assess whether she has a mental illness', 'to discover if there is an organic reason for their behaviour', as if psychiatry holds some sort of ultimate truth about the biology of children's mental-health problems, that other mental-health professionals cannot quite reach. The courts routinely ask for psychiatric assessments giving them much higher status than assessments done by any other mental-health professionals. When I do court reports jointly with other professionals, who often know the case much better than I do, the courts, solicitors or agency requesting the report often continue to correspond with myself as if the report was only written by me.

'A's admission to hospital

After a 2-week treatment supervised by an imam which included rituals, prayer, diet, rest and stopping all contact outside the immediate family, the imam told 'A' and his family that the djinn had been expelled. In his elation 'A', feeling much better, resumed what he believed to be his mission in life (to serve Allah and spread word about Islam). He went out to try and engage passers by in discussions about Islam. A few days later whilst trying to talk to a passer-by about Islam, this particular passer-by punched 'A' and a fight developed. The police were called and decided that 'A' was behaving strangely whilst rambling incoherently about being an imam and Islam. They decided to take him to a nearby psychiatric unit for an urgent assessment. 'A' was admitted against his will to an adolescent unit under a section of the mental health act. He was diagnosed as suffering from a manic-depressive illness. There was no interest shown in taking seriously 'A's and his family's interpretation of the recent events. Treatment consisted of anti-psychotic medication and lithium administered against his will along with a touch of psychoeducation. Psychoeducation consisted of sessions mainly for the family during which they were 'educated' about manic-depressive illness. 'A' spent his time in hospital confused, terrorized, in tears and begging to be discharged. This was interpreted by the consultant of the unit as further evidence that 'A' suffered from manic-depressive illness. 'A's family felt equally confused and tearful saying they no longer knew what to believe but couldn't stand seeing how distressed 'A' had become in the unit. When the section lapsed after a month and the unit could no longer detain 'A' against his will, 'A' did not return to the hospital from weekend leave and was lost to follow-up.

At a meeting about our region's contract with an adolescent unit, I mentioned that given the high number of clients from ethnic minorities admitted to this unit, the unit's staff could benefit from some training to develop greater awareness about beliefs and values of different communities. I dared to suggest that sometimes it's necessary to work outside the medical model if culturally appropriate services are to be provided. The consultant for this unit said that he was offended by this and stated very firmly that the unit is a medical unit, provides medical treatment and no one, no matter what their background, should be deprived of the right to receive this.

Chapter 6

Developing multi-perspective approaches

Child and adolescent psychiatry has followed adult psychiatry down the cul-de-sac of a narrow set of historically and culturally conditioned beliefs, that perpetuates the political interests of the elite and marginalizes the experience of many socially disadvantaged groups. For child and adolescent psychiatry to develop in a manner that reflects the cultural diversity and preoccupations of the post-modern world, existing thinking must be challenged from training levels right up to service delivery to allow a more inclusive, user-informed and multi-perspective approach to develop. This will inevitably challenge the current hierarchical set up.

As I hope you have gathered by now, I believe that there are no special experts in human misery and life's problems, rather, I believe that each culture develops its own sets of beliefs, attitudes and practices, that guide its local communities on these issues. In our current, western culture the idea of scientifically developed knowledge and the need to professionalize and expertize everything in the world around us, is the context in which western child and adolescent psychiatry has developed. The current political and economic domination of the western world has, naturally, lent western psychiatry an air of universal authority and a political means by which to dismiss and then take over other belief systems.

'It's not us who are being narrow minded'. Western criticism of east European psychiatry in the cold war era

It's interesting to look at how western psychiatrists have criticized other psychiatric systems as having a conceptualization of mental disorder that makes them vulnerable to abuse. Those same psychiatrists seem not to have noticed how many of their criticisms apply equally to the system in which they have faith and which they clearly believe is scientifically superior. Take east European psychiatry during the cold-war years for example. Many western commentators have accused old east European psychiatry of human-rights abuses, linking the abuse with problems in the way this psychiatric system defined mental illness. They cite problems such as ill-defined boundaries for psychiatric categories, over use of categories such as 'sluggish schizophrenia' and overt use of political issues in defining symptoms such as 'reformist delusions' (Bloch and Reddaway, 1977; Bloch and Chodoff, 1991).

The history of east European psychiatry is, of course, closely linked to the development of the old USSR (Union of Soviet Socialist Republics), none the less its development, style and concepts show a high degree of similarity to the western psychiatry that criticizes it. Prior to the Bolshevik revolution of 1917, Russian psychiatrists were actively campaigning and developing methods for looking after mental patients without using physical restraints (mostly strait-jackets) (Frieden, 1981) and before such methods became the norm in the west. The Bolshevik revolution brought with it many changes to Russian psychiatry. Psychiatrists were one of the first groups of professionals to offer their support to the new government and many of the profession's leading figures quickly stepped into positions of power in the newly created medical administration (Mitskevich, 1969). Thereafter the 'official' historical accounts and academic training textbooks credit S.S. Korsakov with the paternity of the Russian psychiatric profession. Korsakov is attributed with being the leading figure responsible for the development of non-restraint methods of treatment in Russian psychiatric institutions, and it was thanks to him that the introduction of these methods encountered much less resistance in Russia than in the rest of Europe. Korsakov is credited with revolutionizing the practice of psychiatry in Russia and with introducing a new system for developing psychiatric nosology (Babayan, 1985). Once a system for classification of psychiatric disorders was established, Soviet psychiatry (like psychiatry in western countries) expended a great deal of energy attempting to demonstrate its political reliability on one hand and its medical expertise on the other.

After Korsakov, probably the next most influential author in Soviet psychiatry was the pathologist Davydovskii, whose ideas on the concept of disease in psychiatry first appeared in 1962 (Davydovskii, 1962; Davydovskii and Sil-Vestrov, 1966). This corresponded with a period of growing interest in the same concepts in the west (Akhmedzhanov and Lifshits, 1971; Sil-Vestrov, 1968; Aleksakhina, 1968). Davydovskii's views, which strengthened the dominant Soviet psychiatric schools of thought, were strongly biological. He argued that disease is the reaction of an organism to a pathogen, and its form is influenced by such factors as inheritance, age, sex and previous exposure. He believed that social factors could provoke diseases, and social adaptation could be impaired by disease, but that disease is primarily a biological phenomenon (Davydovskii, 1962). The subsequent central themes in Soviet psychiatry of biological adaptation, norms of bodily structure and functioning and of scientific analysis, all echo the dominant 'medical model' approach favoured by most psychiatric authors in the west (e.g. Roth and Kroll, 1986).

As in the west, 'modern' Soviet psychiatry sought to 'tidy up' mental illness by trying to define it in terms of factual criteria and biological functioning, rather than engaging with a debate about the value-laden, socially constructed aspects of psychiatric classification, beliefs and practices (Boorse, 1975; Kendall, 1975).

As in the west, in much of Soviet psychiatric literature, it was generally assumed that mental and physical diseases are essentially similar (Snezhnevsky, 1971; Snezhnevsky and Vartanyan, 1970).

The differences between the Soviet and western systems for classification of mental disorders were relatively minor, the two systems having common philosophical roots in German phenomenology. Even specific symptoms that have been much criticized, such as 'reformist delusions', are not so different to definitions for symptoms in western psychiatry. Reformist delusions have been criticized as leading to a diagnosis based on a single symptom instead of recognizing that psychiatric diagnoses should be based on syndromes (Merskey and Shafran, 1986). However, western psychiatry recognizes a range of monosymptomatic delusional states such as erotomania (delusional belief that someone, often famous, is in love with you) and Othello syndrome (delusional beliefs of infidelity). 'Reformist delusions' have also been criticized for their political content (Merskey and Shafran, 1986), yet in western psychiatry delusions with political themes are also widely encountered and recognized in a variety of diagnoses. The idea that an experience is a delusion reflects a psychiatric belief that a delusion is an idea expressed by a patient that they (the psychiatrist) believe is culturally atypical. Most Soviet psychiatrists seemed to have believed that, while mistakes are always possible, a majority of those people whom the west called dissidents and who had been diagnosed as mentally ill, were in fact mentally ill (Schmidt *et al.*, 1973).

Thus, like western psychiatry, Soviet psychiatry was attempting to define mental health in medical, biological terms rather than social terms. Like the west, the social-value-laden nature of the system was easily apparent to outsiders (Fulford *et al.*, 1993). In such a system, the interpretive nature of evaluating the client becomes a big factor in determining outcome and treatment. This in turn lends any psychiatric system for classification to become a collection of social, moral, cultural and political judgements. As Kopelman (1990) has argued, the more the evaluative element in a diagnosis is contentious, the greater the scope for abuse, particularly if the subjective nature of evaluation is not acknowledged. Thus in both systems, psychiatry pretending to be an objective science-based practice, has, in effect, been used by the state to successfully marginalize dissenting voices and support 'official' versions of what 'normal' thinking and behaviour should be.

The lack of multi-perspectives in child and adolescent psychiatry

The lessons for the younger profession of child and adolescent psychiatry are clear. Going down a primarily medical biological route is not only scientifically unsound but, more importantly, could lead to the development of a professional culture that has the potential for abusive practices (as in adult psychiatry). To miss and misunderstand the evaluative nature of our diagnosis and interventions sets us down a social, morally, politically and ethically dangerous path. Instead of engaging in debate about our socially value-laden constructs, the effort at present is to increase diagnostic certainty by increasing consensus (i.e. tidying up). The huge possible impacts of this short-sightedness are already apparent (e.g. drug-addict children are created by over-medication, other systems are let off the hook by labelling a problem as medical, a 'psychiatric' career is created for young children by labelling them as suffering from a life-long disorder, genetic eugenic ideas are used to eradicate the growing tide of childhood psychiatric diagnosis). We are, armed with such professional beliefs, condoning ever-narrower definitions of 'normal' for childhood behaviour and child-rearing practices. What I believe we must do in child and adolescent psychiatry, is to start to engage in important and absent conceptual debates. We must acknowledge the limitations of the medical model in our field, challenge the current hierarchical status of western child-psychiatric concepts and allow more diverse voices and perspectives to be heard so that a more multi-perspective approach can develop.

Getting socially marginalized voices into the mainstream is a difficult, complicated, uphill task. The process of training indoctrinates the trainee into a particular belief system. Sadly this means the 'therapization' and 'westernization' of many non-western professionals, who are effectively cultured into a way of thinking that has the potential for distancing them from their own cultural models, before they are allowed back to work with members of their own community. I recall a conversation with a trainee family therapist who had grown up in a Chinese community in Hong Kong and was now training in the UK. She told me how, in a session with a Chinese family (that was being observed and supervised by a white European supervisor), she had a strong wish to talk about food with this family, knowing its central importance to Chinese families. However, she stopped herself because a voice in her head was telling her that this would not be viewed as therapeutic.

When I worked in the very ethnically diverse east London, I often held discussions with health and allied professionals about the role and importance of traditional and spiritual healers to the ethnic-minority community. The differences in the reactions I got, I felt, illustrated the way western professional training can distance people from their own background. When I spoke with the 'untherapized' interpreters and health advocates about the role and importance of traditional and spiritual healers, they spoke at length about how many members of their own community felt the local psychiatric services to be belittling and distrusting, and how often they used traditional and spiritual healers instead. Many also told their own personal stories of cures or help from such practitioners. In contrast, when speaking with trained nurses and social workers with an ethnic-minority background, the responses were much more muted and cautious with many viewing the challenge as being that of educating the local community about mental illness and about the potential dangers of these healers.

Academics too, even those who profess to be interested in ethnic minorities, have the same difficulty accommodating non-mainstream voices. I have sat in an all-white, middle-class, management group consisting of academic psychiatrists, psychologists and others, who were organizing a study day about mental-health issues in refugee families. The day consisted of white clinicians and academics talking about their views concerning refugee families and mental health (which inevitably involved trauma and pathology and the need for more, presumably western style, services). There was not one speaker who was a refugee, nor had any refugee organizations been consulted or invited to take part. I have been invited to take part in a large research project based in east London, coordinated by a professor of psychiatry, which examined the beliefs (with regard to mental health) of second-generation Asian adolescents. The proposal developed by white clinicians suggested that this particular group were ill informed about mental illness and it was hoped that the findings would lead to a programme of education about mental illness that could be carried out in local schools, colleges and media. No interest was shown in what us professionals might learn from this group's ideas and beliefs, in other words how this group might be able to educate us, the professionals. Needless to say, I declined the offer to participate.

Developing multi-perspective approaches

The mental health industry for childhood and adolescence is in danger of killing off and stifling diversity. I believe that we need to take off the shackles of a rigid faith if we are to tap into the creativity that a flexible multi-framework approach can offer. No one person or approach has the definitive answer. Knowledge in the field of child and adolescent mental health is socially constructed, with many valid ways in which we can understand the thinking and behaviour of children and their parents available. The knowledge we use should be seen as culturally informed and situated in ever-changing local contexts and relationships. Professionally invented ideas about these human situations and relationships can be viewed as potentially useful ways (among many others) of thinking about clients' concerns, rather than as objective, empirically verifiable truths. Approached from this angle, the emphasis in our thinking shifts from the search for objectivity and certainty towards a greater engagement with intersubjectivity and curiosity. Rather than imposing expertly given, authoritative, complete and definitive accounts, we can open up alternative perspectives, particularly non-pathological ones that build on strengths and the client's own resources. Child and adolescent psychiatry doesn't need to hide behind the cloak of objective science (Dell, 1982), instead it would benefit from reflecting on its own cultural biases in the definitions and interventions it promotes. It requires a kind of paradigm shift that allows for alternative frames to be used in a way that can bring fresh thinking into a problem. As Watzlawick et al. (1974) point out, our experience of the world is based on the categorization of the objects of our perception into classes and that once an object is conceptualized as the member of a given class, it is extremely difficult to see it as belonging to another class. However, once we can see 'alternative class membership', it becomes difficult to go back to our previously limited view of reality.

Peoples ideas, thoughts and behaviours cannot be understood apart from their socio-cultural contexts (Parre, 1995). For example, to label a housewife as having a 'dependent personality disorder', isolates her from all other women struggling with this issue in contemporary western society and obscures how these characteristics are fostered and encouraged by prevailing gender expectations (Hare-Mustin, 1987; Goldner, 1988; Weingarten, 1994, 1995). Likewise childhood psychiatric labels are in constant danger of defining a child's character in a narrow tunnel vision, stripped of context. Our professional attitude and techniques leave us in constant danger of thoughtlessness about differences in culture, race, gender, class, sexuality and family lifestyle, and of neglecting the impact of the wider system that children live in. Incorporating this 'big-picture' thinking should affect how we conduct our assessments and treatments of children and their families. We need to recognize our fallibility. We need to be concerned with discovering the real strengths of our clients position(s), as participants equally capable of illuminating the subject matter (Warnke, 1987). We need to be able to get closer to the client's language and worldview rather than using the terminology of our own treatment models (Miller *et al.*, 1995). We need to pay greater attention to and even privilege the small and ordinary in conversations with clients (Weingarten, 1998). We need to understand that we cannot be objective outsiders in our dealings with our clients, we are subject to the same world-making and unmaking processes as everyone else (Weingarten, 1998).

In developing our clinical practice to adapt to the post-modern environment and the reality of multicultural society we need to develop a new direction for mental health and to re-examine the goals of psychiatric practice (Bracken and Thomas, 2001). Contexts, that is to say social, political and cultural realities, should become central to our understanding of the conditions we deal with. Practical, clinical, mental-health interventions do not have to be based solely on an individualistic framework and centred on medical diagnosis and treatment. This does not negate the importance of a biological perspective at times but it does mean refusing to privilege this approach. It also means acknowledging that the approaches currently privileged are based on sets of assumptions that are, themselves, derived from a particular context. An ethical rather than technological orientation should be privileged. Because our work is primarily concerned with beliefs, moods, relationships and behaviours, the bulk of our clinical work is underpinned by concepts, values and assumptions rather than a technological evidence base. This means engaging with our clients in discussion about risks as much as it does in engaging in discussion about benefit. It means ending, once and for all, our wish to uncouple mental-health care from debates about culture, power and social exclusion. It means rehabilitating the wisdom of other belief systems' approaches to helping people in a way that can only enhance our flexibility, creativity and therapeutic competence.

Medical anthropologists have already provided some useful ideas that can help us incorporate other systems of thinking into our western-psychiatric approach, some of which I have detailed below.

Symbolic healing

A number of anthropologists have attempted to synthesize cross-cultural theories and ethnographic data about healing practices into a model of how symbolic healing works (Douglas, 1970b; Dow, 1986; Glick, 1967; Horton, 1967; Janzen, 1978; Kleinman and Song, 1979; Messing, 1968; Moerman, 1979; Nash, 1967; Tambiah, 1968; Turner, 1967; Wallace, 1959; Young, 1977; Kleinman, 1988). In summarizing the views that emerge Kleinman (1988) proposes that four structural processes are essential to accomplish symbolic healing.

In stage one a symbolic bridge between personal experience, social relations and cultural meaning is built. The experiences of individuals in society are taken to be signs whose meanings link up with a group's main cultural symbols (e.g. yin/ yang, the crucified Christ or the body/self as a broken machine). These symbols are seen as representing the cultural 'grammar' governing how a person orientates themselves to the world around them.

Stage two commences when this symbolic connection is activated for a particular person. This person then seeks out a healer to help them. The healer then persuades this person that the problem from which they are suffering can be redefined in terms of the system of cultural meaning that predominates (e.g. hallucinations could be seen as the work of the Devil and therefore to be treated by exorcism). Matters proceed smoothly if the healer, the patient, their family and the community are in agreement about the core meanings of the presenting problem.

In stage three the healer then skilfully guides therapeutic change in the person's emotional reactions through mediating symbols taken from that culture's general belief system. These symbols are often then manipulated in healing rituals (e.g. the Navaho singers' images of the sacred mountains).

In stage four the healer confirms the transformation of the symbols (e.g. the invading spirit, now named and understood, has been subject to specific rituals of exorcism, or the oedipal conflict now understood is worked through in the interpretation of personal events and the experience of transference to the therapist). In this final stage the healing interaction has been turned into a meaningful experience resulting in the affirmation of success.

In this model of healing the healer (whatever their orientation) is encouraging emotional distancing and release by using culturally meaningful mediating symbols. The emotional change can alter the patient's cognition and as a result their social relationships. The restructuring of social relationships, a key feature of healing rituals in non-western societies and sometimes an unintended part of western psychotherapy intensifies the process of transforming cognition.

Unfortunately, these healing processes, which in effect illustrate how deeply intuitive and psychologically minded most non-western cultures are, have become increasingly marginal to the west's dominant healing systems. Psychiatry has essentially followed the trend in biomedicine where research on disease has been given a higher priority than the care of the patient (Sullivan, 1986). All too often this has encouraged medical approaches to patient care that are not only ineffective but are also considered by many to be inhumane (Eisenberg and Kleinman, 1981). Talk therapies and the non-specific (placebo) use of symbols are disdained. Yet most of the psychiatrist's work is about people's life stories, their aspirations, their joy, their passions and tragedies. It unavoidably has to do with those deeply personal and life-world problem issues. Yet psychiatry continues to be under pressure to become another version of high-technology medicine. Although the practice of psychotherapy continues to thrive, particularly in the private sector because of consumer demands, the psychiatrists' concern with symbolic trans-formations is getting less and less attention in medical schools, teaching hospitals and training rotations.

Child psychiatrists, like adult psychiatrists, are being told by the influential neuropsychiatric (as if such a thing exists) lobby, that psychiatrists should leave psychosocial enquiry and therapy to other categories of health professionals such as nurses, psychologists and social workers. One would think that not only every psychiatrist, but every medical student too, should be trained to elicit the highest rates of placebo effects and develop their mastery of non-specific symbolic tech-niques. Unfortunately, medical students are taught little else than that placebos confound clinical trials and it may be unethical to provide them without the consent of the patient. Biomedicine is the major system of healing used in the west, yet it has little to do with what is most central to most healing systems – symbolic healing (Kleinman, 1988). The inevitable effect of this trend is a curtailment of our therapeutic ability and efficiency.

The psychiatrist as cultural interpreter

We are always interpreting each other whether we are psychiatrists, therapists or clients, or just talking to each other in the course of our daily lives. All too often we confuse our values, beliefs and practices with the ultimate truth. When dealing with subjective reality without material facts we are dealing with representations of reality. 'The map is not the territory', as Bateson (1973) noted. A representation describes the way something is believed to be and there can be many competing or complementary representations, just as one word or symbol may have many meanings. In order to understand the speech and acts of others we must understand something about their social relations, social conditions and cultural beliefs. This process of making meaning of other people's lives is a challenge to any kind of therapeutic process, but particularly so where an obvious cultural difference is present between the therapist and the client (Krause, 1998). There has never been and never will be any human activity which is devoid of meaning and these meanings can never be fixed into a concrete state by a 'trick' of classification. Furthermore, we are never detached observers in our work and we must accept ourselves as active participants in the therapeutic contexts we create.

According to some, one of the first conditions for responsible and sensitive practice is for the therapist to recognize their own position within the system (Cecchin, 1987; Jones, 1995; Hardham, 1996). Whenever we encounter difference to ourselves, even to a minor degree, these differences are understood and conceptualized in relation to ourselves (Bateson, 1973, 1979). Whether this is overtly acknowledged by the practitioner is an important matter and if the above ideas have any validity then sensitive and responsible therapists of all persuasions must be capable of a disciplined search into the cultural assumptions that they bring into any therapeutic encounter. In other words it is not enough to simply enquire about the differences between a client's beliefs, lifestyle and practices and your own, as if your own beliefs and values are the norms against which the client's should be judged. It means being able to acquire some appreciation of why clients come to do what they do, of why they are participants in their own contexts and of how they understand themselves (Taylor, 1985). It also means trying to understand how we, as psychiatrists, have come to believe what we believe and how our beliefs and practices will impact on the process of therapy between ourselves and our clients.

If the psychiatrist is able to engage at least partially with this question of differences to our clients and the assumptions that we take into our therapy sessions, then a more equal and therapeutically useful form of communication can take place. If it is only the psychiatrist who is setting the agenda, then an inequality or overt imbalance in power can still result in questions receiving an answer, but these answers may well teach the psychiatrist more about their own preoccupations than those of the clients.

For a therapist or psychiatrist to become truly successful in developing a therapeutic level of communication, they should be able to work outside the constraints of a theoretical framework in a way that allows a continuous stimulation of their curiosity; the sort of curiosity that is often inhibited by ideology-driven frameworks. Indeed, as I have discussed in the preceding chapters, theory is embedded in social, political and cultural matrices. Thus, because theory can become so ideologically driven, the psychiatrist needs to be able to, from time to time, turn theories upside down so that all the assumptions within a theory about what is normal and deviant can become a topic for questioning and curiosity again. The more I encounter difference the more I find my notions of what is universal changing. As I mentioned in Chapter 2, I am not arguing that there are no universals but I am saying that the apparent universals that psychiatric practice would have us believe exist are open to question. What we have are value judgements that we impose upon others. Questioning these universals means questioning these value systems in a way that allows us to listen to clients' value systems in a less judgemental way.

Coming from Iraq a year earlier than my parents when I was 14 years old was my 'normal'. Of course, there were elements of that time that I found distressing, upsetting and confusing. Yet there were also things that I found exciting and educational. I came to believe that this experience was psychologically traumatic as those around me in this country, and then my therapist, interpreted my experience as traumatic. The things that I experienced as difficult during this year (e.g. the difference in peer-group attitudes towards girls and the verbal teasing about being an Arab) were not necessarily the same as the things that the representatives of this culture, such as my therapist, interpreted as traumatic (e.g. the separation from my parents).

In essence what all of us who are working in the field of therapy for social suffering are doing is acting as cultural interpreters. We give meaning to our clients' utterances and actions through the use of an interpretive frame. If both client and therapist share an interpretive framework then the symbolic healing process described above can proceed relatively smoothly. If we have little understanding of the client's cultural framework then modern, western psychiatry will still impose its own interpretations. Then the psychiatrist, rather than acting as a skilful, cultural interpreter, will act as a clumsy, cultural colonizer. If, on the other hand, the psychiatrist has become adept at moving in and out of different frameworks of meaning, at trying to understand the client's own interpretive framework and at searching for symbolic meanings that can transform and change situations in a positive manner, then the psychiatrist can become a competent, cultural interpreter, a competent agent of therapeutic change, a competent psychiatrist.

Much of what I have said above reflects what some might call a post-modern attitude to child and adolescent psychiatry (and psychiatry in general). I discuss some particular post-modern therapeutic techniques (such as solution-focused and narrative therapy) in Chapter 8. This opening up of the meaning systems we use that I am proposing would be a massive challenge to the institution of child and adolescent psychiatry that has come to be controlled by the rigid ideological dogma of biomedicine. However, changes in the way our profession thinks about its subject matter are unavoidable if child psychiatry wishes to avoid further damning criticism and wishes to contribute towards developing services that are both culturally appropriate and geared towards the best interests of children.

Alternatives for 'A's treatment

If only the adolescent boy 'A' from my example in Chapter 3 had been listened to. If only the adolescent unit he was admitted to was not so concerned with imposing its manic-depression medical model and had taken the family's story seriously. If only the consultant for the unit had been brave enough to wonder if 'A' and his family's interpretation of events had as much, if not more, relevance than his/her own symptom-derived ones. A real window of opportunity could have opened up. A conversation on the lines of 'you are understandably high and elated after getting rid of the djinn' could have taken place. 'A's experiences could have been validated instead of crushed as meaningless. The role of the adolescent unit (if any) could have been framed very differently: 'after such a difficult few months in your life, you may need a bit of time to recuperate and build up your strength' as opposed to the 'you are here to be treated for your illness'. Conversations with 'A' and his family, that included comments on their loyalty, dedication to each other, their ability to actively seek solutions, to survive adverse experiences and so on, could have taken place. A lack of knowledge about Islam, djinn-possession states and the family's cultural background could have been admitted to. This may have led to some helpful empowering conversations with the family and 'A' (where they are effectively the experts). It may have led to active use of an interpreter or health advocate for information and advice about culturally appropriate interventions. It may even have led to consultations with a local imam or the imam who had carried out the treatment for 'A' (if they could be persuaded to trust a western psychiatric professional).

In his personal account of recovery from psychosis, May (2000) discusses how going through the psychiatric system (including recurrent admission to hospital) left him with an overwhelming sense of being undervalued. He was helped by a friend of his who seemed to believe that the situation was something he could 'get over'. He also recalled the importance of family stories about making a better than expected recovery from a serious illness as a child and how other children used to trust him and tell him their problems. He was also helped by remembering a comment that 'this boy will do well' from one of his teachers at primary school. He felt he had to hold on to these more positive stories, as an alternative to the hope-killing 'you'll be mentally ill for the rest of your life' story he was getting from the medical professionals.

Chapter 7

The case of attention deficit hyperactivity disorder (ADHD)

Some years ago I attended a conference organized by a pro-Ritalin® and pro-ADHD group. At this conference I heard an American professor talk about his 'success' stories in treating adults with Ritalin®. He spoke about a high-flying lawyer who complained he couldn't concentrate in meetings. The professor prescribed Ritalin® and the lawyer was delighted at his improved ability to concentrate. I heard a prominent paediatrician tell us that most problems of childhood, adolescence and young adulthood (such as substance misuse, behavioural problems, delinquency, depression, learning difficulties, bullying, poor peer relationships, poor academic achievement and so on) were caused by untreated ADHD. I heard about Ritalin® and other psychostimulants spoken of in terms of miracles and complete transformations, and the terms revolutionary, state-of-the-art and hugely under-prescribed were frequently used. I didn't hear any mention of the risks or controversies associated with prescribing psychostimulants. Non-believers were spoken about in a derogatory manner as if their concerns amounted to blasphemy. I left the conference feeling that I had attended an extremist cult convention, not a scientific conference.

I decided to buy Green and Chee's (1997) book *Understanding ADHD: a parent's Guide to Attention Deficit Hyperactivity Disorder in Children* having seen many parents refer to this book. I read that parents with children who have ADHD say things like 'what I tell him goes in one ear and out of the other', 'with homework I get nowhere unless I stand over him', 'he's impossible in the morning', 'he can remember details of what happened to him last year but forgets what I said 2 minutes ago', 'he doesn't seem to learn from experience', 'he has no road sense', 'he's got such a short fuse', 'she was such a demanding baby she took up every minute of my life', 'this toddler is constantly on the move', 'she hates to be restricted, she loves to be outside' and so on. I couldn't understand this. The book was describing my and, I reckon, most parents' children. Why were these extremely common behaviours (particularly amongst boys) being listed as if they were signs of what the book refers to as a 'biological, brain-based condition' (Green and Chee, 1997: 2). I wonder what I would have thought on reading this if I were a parent who was worried about my child's behaviour or development?

I began to think about the 'big picture' here. What was this all about? It dawned on me that the concept of ADHD was intimately tied up with our modern, western beliefs about childhood and child rearing. Social pressures build up certain expectations for children to live up to. Parents (and other guardians such as teachers) feel blamed when their children cannot be squeezed into a socially desirable shape. Doctors, as powerful priests of knowledge, then define this problem medically and, hey presto, a gravy train starts running for the multi-million dollar pharmaceutical industry.

But is all this medicalization desirable? I guess it has helped some individuals. But then I see boy after boy coming to my clinics who have been diagnosed and medicated for years. I see boy after boy who hate taking these medicines. I discuss the controversies with the parents and nearly all want to reduce the dose or bring their children off these tablets. I've seen boy after boy come off psychostimulants. Parents tell me their child started eating normally again, put on weight, came out of their shell and began to express themselves again. They were transformed (as a pro-Ritalin® advocate might say). I wondered what those years on medication were doing to their brains and bodies for such dramatic changes to be noticed. I wondered if this is another Valium® story in the making. I wondered how many of my colleagues discuss the controversies and air both sides of the story with their clients. I wondered how many parents are routinely denied the information about risks that is needed to make a properly informed choice. I wondered if this individualized medicalization of a child is a sign that many doctors have completely forgotten what a community is. I wondered if the problem is this apparent enormous rise in the number of boys suffering from a medical condition or is it a growing problem in the system or society that manages them.

A cultural history of attention deficit hyperactivity disorder

Overactivity, poor concentration and impulsivity in children were first conceptualized as medical phenomena earlier this century. The first recorded interest in children with poor attention and hyperactivity dates back to the turn of the century when a paediatrician, Frederick Still, described a group of children who showed an abnormal incapacity for sustained attention, restlessness and fidgetiness, and went on to argue that these children had deficiencies in volitional inhibition (Still, 1902). Hyperactivity and poor attention in children then came to be viewed as being linked when the diagnosis of minimal brain damage was coined. The idea of minimal brain damage had originally gained favour following epidemics of encephalitis in the first decades of the twentieth century. Post-encephalitic children often presented with restlessness, personality changes and learning difficulties. Then came a chance discovery in the 1930s that psychostimulant medication could reduce the restlessness, hyperactivity and behavioural problems that these children presented with (Bradley, 1937). This gave rise to early theories about organic lesions in the brain causing hyperactivity and poor attention in other children and so led to the invention of the minimal brain damage diagnosis. Strauss's writings in the 1940s (e.g. Strauss and Lehtinen, 1947) strengthened this idea further by suggesting that hyperactivity, in the absence of a family history of subnormality, should be considered as sufficient evidence for a diagnosis of brain damage. By the 1960s, however, the term minimal brain damage was losing favour because evidence for underlying organic lesions in children who displayed poor attention and overactivity was not being found. Instead there was a growing interest in behaviourally defined syndromes. Despite the abandonment of the minimal brain damage hypothesis the assumption that this syndrome does indeed have a discoverable and specific physical cause, related to some sort of brain dysfunction, survived in the new behaviourally-based definition. Yet studies have shown that demonstrable minimal brain damage from a variety of causes, predisposes the child to the development of a wide range of psychiatric diagnosis as opposed to a particular type such as ADHD (Schmidt *et al.*, 1987).

So it was that in the mid-1960s the US-based *Diagnostic and Statistical Manual of Mental Disorders* second edition (DSM-II), coined the label 'hyperkinetic reaction of childhood', to replace the diagnosis of minimal brain damage (Sandburg, 1996). Over the following three decades this new behaviourally defined condition rose from being a matter of peripheral interest in child psychiatric practice and research in North America to a place of central prominence.

The second edition, DSM-II, was replaced in the early 1980s by the third edition, DSM-III (American Psychiatric Association, 1980). The disorder was now termed attention deficit disorder (ADD). This could be diagnosed with or without hyper-activity and was defined using three dimensions (three separate lists of symptoms); one for attention deficit, one for impulsivity and one for hyperactivity. The three-dimensional approach was abandoned in the late 1980s when DSM-III was revised, becoming DSM-III-R (American Psychiatric Association, 1987), in favour of combining all the symptoms into one list (one dimension). The new term for the disorder was attention deficit hyperactivity disorder (ADHD), with attention, hyperactivity and impulsiveness now assumed to be part of one disorder with no distinctions. When the fourth edition of DSM, DSM-IV (American Psychiatric Association, 1994), reconsidered the diagnosis the criteria were again changed, this time in favour of a two-dimensional model with attention deficit being one sub-category and hyperactivity and impulsiveness the other. With each revision a larger cohort of children is found to be above the threshold for diagnosis. For example, changing from DSM-III to DSM-III-R more than doubled the number of children from the same population who were diagnosed with the disorder (Lindgren *et al.*, 1994). Changing from DSM-III-R to DSM-IV increased the prevalence by a further two thirds, with the criteria now having the potential to diagnose the vast majority of children with academic or behavioural problems in a school setting (Baumgaertel *et al.*, 1995). Indeed, according to DSM-IV, the diagnosis 'ADHD not otherwise specified' should be made if there are prominent symptoms of inattention or hyperactivity and impulsivity that do not meet the full ADHD criteria (DSM-IV, American Psychiatric Association, 1994). If we were to interpret this concretely (as doctors often do) it suggests that nearly all children (particularly boys) at some time in their lives could meet one of the definitions and warrant a diagnosis of ADHD.

In the UK child psychiatrists have, in the past, generally followed the diagnostic guidelines of the International Classification of Diseases (ICD) in preference to DSM. The latest edition of ICD (ICD-10, World Health Organization, 1990) has a more explicit definition of hyperkinetic disorder than its predecessor, ICD-9. In common with the trend in DSM revisions, centres that have changed from using ICD-9 to ICD-10 criteria, have also noticed that the diagnosis is being made more frequently (Steinhausen and Erdin, 1991). However, practice in the UK is now moving towards using ADHD as the diagnosis in preference to hyperkinetic syndrome thereby following the terminology used in American practice. Along with Coca-Cola, McDonalds and Hollywood, domination of the world's markets allows American culture to be successfully exported. An enthusiastic drug industry and drug-industry-funded pro-Ritalin® parent groups, helped establish ADHD as the main diagnostic label to use. This is evident from the fact that clinics being set up in this country, both private and National Health Service clinics, call themselves ADHD clinics as opposed to hyperkinetic disorder clinics. Titles used in publications, media reports and academic conferences commonly refer to ADHD. Attention deficit hyperactivity disorder has taken over as the main term being used.

A leap of faith

So what is the evidence for the existence of this disorder? Is there a medical test that will diagnose it? No. Are there any specific cognitive, metabolic or neurological markers for ADHD? No. Attention deficit hyperactivity disorder is a cultural construct diagnosed on the basis of clinical opinion and faithful belief of the practitioner and is often presented as if it were a biological fact. Those who have argued that ADHD does not exist as a real disorder start by pointing to the obvious uncertainty about its definition (McGuinness, 1989). Indeed, despite years of work and billions of dollars spent on research, the validity of ADHD or hyperkinetic disorder as a disorder distinct from other types of behavioural disturbances in childhood, particularly those involving aggressive and defiant behaviours, has not been established (Prior and Sanson, 1986; Werry et al., 1987a, 1987b). Thus, because of the uncertainty about definition it is hardly surprising that epidemiological studies have produced very different prevalence rates for ADHD or hyperkinetic disorders, ranging from about 0.5 per cent to about 17 per cent of school-age children (Taylor and Hemsley, 1995; Szatmari et al., 1989a).

Epidemiological studies have found a preponderance of boys over girls in ADHD symptomatology, in the region of four (or more) boys to one girl (McGee et al., 1992). This is very similar to the gender distribution found in conduct disorder and other so called externalizing behavioural disorders in children. The meaning of this gender distribution never seems to be questioned. What sort of biological variable are we attempting to categorize here if this is a biological abnormality? Is it that boys generally have bad genes compared to girls? Is it something to do with the normal biological differences between male and female genes? Is there an interaction between boys' behaviour and changes in social expectations regarding children's behaviour generally? Do social changes in family structure, lifestyles, teaching methods, classroom sizes, rates of violence, rates of substance misuse and so on have an effect on perceptions and beliefs about boys' and girls' behaviour, or even on their behaviour directly? Has life got harder for boys in some way? Has life got harder for parents trying to control normal boy behaviour? Are we still compelled to pay more attention to the externalized behaviour of boys than to the internalized behaviour of girls, only now we medicalize this (after all adults in western societies are usually more tolerant of hyperactivity in girls than in boys (Battle and Lacey, 1972))? Do changes in teaching methods and a predominance of female teachers have an effect on how we understand and deal with boys' behaviour? These and other social and cultural questions are never discussed in the medical literature. The gender distribution problem has led some researchers to try and bypass this clear, cultural, construct problem by rather creatively suggesting that biologically the same disorder may present as attention deficit without hyperactivity in girls, thereby evening out the gender ratio (Lahey *et al.*, 1994).

Despite attempts at standardizing criteria and assessment tools in cross-cultural studies, major and significant differences between raters from different countries continue to be apparent (Mann *et al.*, 1992). For example, a cross-cultural study examining clinicians' ratings of the same video tapes of hyperactive and antisocial children (Prendergast *et al.*, 1988) showed that British child and adolescent psychiatrists in the study tended to give more weight to antisocial features and select a diagnosis of conduct disorder, whereas their American colleagues paid attention to hyperactivity signs and identified a primary hyperactivity disorder more readily. It was suggested in this paper that the difference in prevalence between the two countries was an issue of diagnostic practice, training and attitude, not a true epidemiological difference. My point is, however, that these categories are cultural constructs in the first instance and therefore whatever constructs you have grown to believe in, will naturally lead you to focus in that direction. This example of two groups of psychiatrists is interesting as it seems to show that the different belief systems that the psychiatrists held led to a different focus when it came to observing the same sets of behaviours, and therefore a different diagnostic conclusion. I am not suggesting that one is better than the other, but simply making the point that both are culturally constructed belief systems. This is further confirmed when you look at clinical practice within a country. For example, Rappley *et al.* (1995) found that the rate of diagnosis of ADHD varied by a factor of ten from county to county within the same state (in the US). There are also significant differences between raters when they rate children from different ethnic minority backgrounds (Sonuga-Barke *et al.*, 1993). One replicated finding is an apparently high rate of hyperactivity in China and Hong Kong (Shen *et al.*, 1985; Luk and Leung, 1989). In these studies nearly three times as many Chinese as English children were rated as hyperactive. A more detailed assessment of these results suggested that most of the 'hyperactive' Chinese children would not have been rated as hyperactive by most English raters and were a good deal less hyperactive than the English children rated as 'hyperactive' (Taylor, 1994). One suggestion for such a consistently large disparity in hyperactivity ratings between Chinese and English children, is that it may be because of the great importance of school success in Chinese culture, leading to an intolerance of much lesser degrees of disruptive behaviour (Taylor, 1994). Whatever the reason(s), it demonstrates that hyperactivity and disruptiveness in boys is a highly culturally constructed entity.

That ratings of hyperactivity, inattention and disruptiveness are highly culturally dependent is not surprising as inattention, impulsivity and motor restlessness are found in all children (and adults) to some degree. Diagnosis is based on an assessment of what is felt to be developmentally inappropriate intensity, frequency and duration of the behaviours, rather than on its mere presence. All the symptoms described in this disorder are of a subjective nature (e.g. 'often does not seem to listen when spoken to') and therefore highly influenced by the raters' cultural beliefs and perceptions about such behaviours. After all, how do you operationalize, define and understand non-specific words like 'often', which are invariably found in ADHD-rating questionnaires?

Then there is the whole thorny question of comorbidity. Numerous epidemio-logical and clinical studies demonstrate the high frequency with which supposedly separate child psychiatric disorders occur in individuals with ADHD (Caron and Rutter, 1991). In children with ADHD comorbidity with other child psychiatric conditions is common no matter what definition is used (Biederman et al., 1991). It is estimated that about half the children with ADHD also have a conduct disorder, about half have an emotional disorder, about one third have an anxiety disorder and another third have major depression (Barkley, 1994). Comorbidity is so prevalent that nearly all ADHD-diagnosed children will have at least one other diagnosable child-psychiatric condition (Hazell, 1997). The co-occurrence of the symptoms that make up oppositional defiant and conduct disorders with those that make up hyperactivity and attention deficit disorders is so strong (Biederman et al., 1991; Fergusson and Horwood, 1993; Fergusson et al., 1991; Szatmari et al., 1989b) that many commentators have questioned the reality of the distinction between them (Hinshaw, 1987). What does this all mean?

I think that the concept of comorbidity has been adopted by psychiatrists as a way of trying to explain clinical reality when it does not appear to tally with research-generated views of mental life. It's a way of maintaining a fantasy that there is a natural, probably biological, boundary where no natural boundaries exist (Tyrer, 1996). This may be because in conditions such as ADHD, like many other psychiatric diagnoses, the extent to which neuronal circuits in the brain are involved vary individually and do not have an obvious one-to-one causal relationship with the psychiatric diagnoses (Van Praag, 1996). In other words, if or when we get to the stage where we are able to do reliable tests to pick up some sort of chemical imbalance in the brain, we may well find that there is no obvious correspondence between say (for the sake of argument) a dopamine imbalance and the symptoms of ADHD. Some children with a dopamine imbalance will have symptoms of ADHD, which may well be causally related to this imbalance, and others with ADHD won't (and therefore in these children dopamine imbalance couldn't be causally related). Furthermore the massive amounts of comorbidity present suggests that our current diagnostic framework does not reflect a coherent medically based one, related to physical biological causes. To take up my example of a dopamine imbalance again, this means that among children suffering from a dopamine imbalance in one child this imbalance may cause ADHD-type symptoms, in another it may cause more anxiety-type symptoms, in another it may cause a mixture of ADHD-type and depressive-type symptoms, in another it may cause no symptoms and so on. In such a scenario, the current diagnostic system would, in a medical sense, become redundant; instead we would have a more physically valid diagnosis (e.g. dopamine imbalance syndrome) and a medical way of establishing the physical component to a mental-health problem. Furthermore, we would have a clear rational scientific basis for the physical component of any treatment and for building coherent, scientific, research-based knowledge of this physical component. Only when there is a clear test to establish this physical component is a medical linear argument valid. Until then, in any individual child, it is pure speculation. Castles built on sand. If the foundation assumption is wrong the castle collapses. In that sense our current so-called knowledge base is no different to, say, a religious knowledge base and no more or less valid.

This lack of a coherent concept is reflected in the lack of consensus on the question of possible causal mechanisms. Thus the condition was initially viewed as being due to an underlying, excessive motor activity in the child (Schachar, 1986) and later as being due to an underlying central attention deficit (Douglas, 1972, 1983). Others have suggested that the central deficit is one of generalized intellectual impairment (Werry et al., 1987a) or of motivation (Draeger et al., 1986). The conviction held by a number of influential researchers about the likely central deficit has had a big influence on the behavioural definitions of the disorder. For example, Douglas's belief (1972) that attention, not hyperactivity, was the essential feature distinguishing these children from other difficult and disruptive children, led to the establishment of the 'attention deficit disorder (ADD)' definition in DSM-III. There is not even consensus on whether the core behaviours (of inattention, impulsivity and hyperactivity) need always be present (i.e. pervasive) or need to be observable in only one situation (e.g. school or home) for a diagnosis to be valid. Some suggest that the behaviours need to be pervasive (e.g. Taylor et al., 1991) and others conclude that pervasiveness is not a necessary condition of a valid definition (e.g. Szatmari et al., 1989a).

Claims have been made that neuroimaging studies have confirmed that ADHD is a brain disorder. Closer examination of the quoted studies reveals a more complex picture. PET (Position Emission Tomography), SPECT (Single Photon Emission Computerized Tomography), EEG (Electroencephelogram) and MRI (Magnetic Resonance Imaging) scan studies have not uncovered a consistent deficit or abnormality, with a wide variety of brain structures being implicated, for example striatal, orbital, prefrontal, frontoposterior and medial orbital areas, caudate nucleus, corpus calosum and parietal lobe (see Rapport, 1995). In none of these neuroimaging studies have the brains of these ADHD children been considered to be clinically abnormal in any way (Hynd and Hooper, 1995). The sample sizes have all been small. The large variety of findings and the inconsistency of results does, I believe, lend support to the above argument that ADHD symptomatology does not have a unique and consistent biological component. What we end up with is speculative 'biobabble'. Even if consistent differences in neuroimaging studies were found, unidirectional cause and effect cannot be assumed if there is an absence of anatomical abnormalities. This is because neurochemical measures may reflect different children's different reactions to the same situation causing differences in brain chemistry, rather than different brain chemistry causing different behaviour (Christie *et al.*, 1995).

As I have argued earlier, what has made diagnosis a useful way of categorizing health problems in the rest of medicine is that the diagnoses point to unique aetiological processes. There is nothing strange about this opinion as many commentators have pointed out that ultimately useful categorizations in medicine are ones that point to unique aetiological processes (Biederman *et al.*, 1991; Klein and Riso, 1994; Taylor, 1988). These unique aetiological processes are completely absent from most psychiatric diagnoses and similarly in ADHD no such processes have been identified, very much the reverse in fact as the evidence above appears to demonstrate. Indeed, the National Institute of Health, a government body in the US, has recently concluded that there is no evidence to support the proposition that ADHD is a biological brain disorder (National Institute of Health, 1998). This conclusion is further supported by a large body of family (Cantwell 1972; Stewart *et al.*, 1980; Welner *et al.*, 1977), twin (Eaves *et al.*, 1993; Gillis *et al.*, 1992; Goodman and Stevenson, 1989; Graham and Stevenson, 1985; Rhee *et al.*, 1995; Stevenson and Graham, 1988; Thapar *et al.*, 1995) and adoption studies (Cantwell, 1975; Cunningham *et al.*, 1975) that support the idea that a genetic component contributes to hyperactivity, conduct disorder and other externalizing behaviours in a manner that suggests a common genetic mechanism underlies all these disorders (Silberg *et al.*, 1996). Presumably this common genetic mechanism has something to do with being boys.

Children described as having ADHD do not appear to have cognitive deficits in attentional mechanisms (Van Der Meere, 1996). The conclusion that children described as having ADHD have inhibitory deficits due to abnormal brain functioning which leads to them performing poorly on standard neuropsychological tests of inhibition, has been undermined by studies that demonstrate that the impulsiveness is reduced when the link between speed of response and the length of the research session is removed (Sonuga-Barke *et al.*, 1994), i.e. when the possibility that these children were getting bored with the experimental test is taken into consideration. A very frequent clinical observation of children with poor concentration and impulsiveness is that this picture changes dramatically when they play their computer games or watch their favourite video, where many so-called ADHD children demonstrate a high ability to concentrate for extended periods of time (another example of typical boy behaviour?).

Most ADHD review articles thus conclude with broad sweeps that have little to offer the clinician in the way of aetiological explanation. For example, Hinshaw (1994: 64) concludes that 'the development of most cases of ADHD is more likely to constitute a complex intertwining of intra individual, familial and broader systems factors than a purely environmental or purely genetic causal route'. Schachar (1991: 181) concludes 'hyperactivity is thought to represent the behavioural manifestation of various underlying psychological, biological and social processes acting singly or in concert'. In a recent review, the British Psychological Society (1996: 24) concludes 'it is probably not useful to think of ADHD as a mental disorder given the current understanding of the psychological basis of the concept'. In the rest of medicine this lack of ability to establish cause would lead to the label 'idiopathic'. Thus a more medically and scientifically accurate label for these children would be 'idiopathic inattention' or 'idiopathic hyperactivity'. Despite the overwhelming evidence that ADHD cannot be conceptualized in a simplistic, linear, unicausal way, authors in influential journals still write completely unsupported statements such as 'attention deficit hyperactivity disorder is a condition of brain dysfunction ... it is a genetic, inherited condition' (Kewley, 1998: 1594). Articles such as this and many others in both the medical and popular press which offer propaganda for an opinion masquerading as fact, contribute to the process of the ADHD construct being passed on from the medical profession to the general public and into general cultural consciousness, as if ADHD were an already understood biological condition.

These conceptual difficulties are no less problematic for those more 'moderate' of believers. In their influential paper 'Recognising hyperactivity: a guide for the cautious clinician', Hill and Cameron (1999) stumble along in a clumsy manner not quite knowing how to conceptualize this construct. Thus they conclude 'in other words a primary hyperactivity disorder is a serious mental health problem, largely biologically determined' (Hill and Cameron, 1999: 52). A couple of pages later they have changed their mind 'hyperactivity is a reflection of an underlying deficit that may have several ultimate causes but a common final path at a behavioural level' (Hill and Cameron, 1999: 54). The serious conceptual problem for the authors of how to separate this apparent multifactorial hyperactivity from this apparent serious biological condition is not tackled.

All those who take part in research and use the diagnosis of ADHD without questioning its basis, have already taken the first leap of faith in accepting that 'there now appears to be little doubt about the validity of the concept' (Toone and Van Der Linden, 1997: 489). Then, in my opinion, there are the religious fanatics like Dr Kewley quoted above. These fundamentalists see ADHD wherever they look. They view ADHD in a cult-like fashion believing it to be a more common than internationally recognized, biological and genetic condition (Kewley, 1999). Dr Kewley believes that this medical illness, when undiagnosed and untreated (primarily by medication), leads to just about every psychosocial problem you could think of, for example criminality, school exclusion, substance misuse, conduct disorder, lack of motivation, learning difficulties, poor self-esteem, depression, obsessionality and so on. He then has the cheek to accuse others of perpetuating 'trite and simplistic explanations for the symptoms of the disorder'! (Kewley, 1999: 18). In *Understanding ADHD: A Parent's Guide to Attention Deficit Hyperactivity Disorder in Children* (Green and Chee, 1997), everything seems to be explained in terms of ADHD. Thus, children with ADHD can be 'superb at sports . . . One of Australia's rugby greats was recently in trouble for impulsive outbursts on the field' (Green and Chee, 1997: 33). On the previous page it is mentioned that children with ADHD are poor at sports because 'they have difficulty in coordinating a sequence of movement' (Green and Chee, 1997: 32). A whole host of social problems are also put down to ADHD 'a common pattern for ADHD disordered men is to conceive then leave' (Green and Chee, 1997: 56) and 'the genes of ADHD predispose families to more restless, mobile, unsettled lifestyles. When I visit the remote mining towns of Australia I see many isolated mothers with challenging children. The busy men folk love the twenty four hour action of the mine' (Green and Chee, 1997: 56). Thus for the fanatics, even context is interpreted as being the result of a biological condition.

Such loose, unsubstantiated and easy option definitions (if only there was a quick diagnosis and instant cure for life's problems!) has many cultural knock-on effects (as well as golden opportunities to make some quick bucks). Rates of diagnosis in the UK have been increasing exponentially over the past decade. Private and National Health Service ADHD clinics are proliferating. It is even possible now to get a diagnosis of ADHD without ever being seen by a professional as some paediatricians, child psychiatrists and educational psychologists in the UK now offer diagnosis over the phone or via the internet (Baldwin and Cooper, 2000).

Fortunately, not everybody associated with the medical profession accepts unquestioningly the trite simplistic explanations put forward by the fundamentalists. For example, Professor Rose of the Brain and Behaviour Research Group with the Open University, referring to ADHD writes

> this sudden emergence of a genetic disorder is puzzling. The result of mass mutations? Scarcely likely . . . All part of the medicalisation of daily life. Naughty and disruptive children have doubtless always existed. In the past their unruly behaviour might have been ascribed to poor parenting, poverty, impoverished schools, or unsympathetic teachers . . . Now we blame the victim instead; there is original sin in them there genes.
>
> (Rose, 1998: 317)

I have deliberately left the issue of medication for later in this chapter.

Cultural models for attention deficit hyperactivity disorder-type behaviours

So ADHD is a cultural construct. But why has it become such a prominent and popular one? What alternative frameworks are there, other than the biological one to give meaning to so-called ADHD behaviours?

I want to suggest that some of the reasons behind the growing interest can be found by looking at the nature of cultural, political and social changes that have occurred in many western countries in the past few decades. Let me start by briefly considering the situation in the US.

Being a parent in the US has become more and more difficult. Issues such as violence, poverty and the breakdown of the family unit have been affecting ever increasing numbers of families (Long, 1996). The index for the social health of the US, which is produced by Fordham University's Institute for Social Policy is based on 16 measures including infant mortality, homicide, teenage suicide, unemployment and drug abuse (Miringoff, 1994). This index gives a score ranging from 0 to 100 (with 100 indicating the best social health). This index has declined from 74 in 1970 to 41 in 1992 indicating growing adversity facing US families. In 1994, there were over 4000 children murdered, over 15 million children living in poverty and over 14 million children living in single-parent families (Children's Defence Fund, 1994). Life has got tougher for US families particularly as you go down in socio-economic status.

The sense of social breakdown and fear of social breakdown in the lives of children in the UK is also evident in the daily recurrent media reports and debates about school crises, discipline problems, expulsion, violence in the young, crime in the young, bullying, drug abuse, break up of the family and breakdown in parent–teacher relationships. A recent study on what was loosely termed psychosocial disorders amongst the young (such as suicide attempts, alcohol and drug abuse, criminality) concluded that there has been a sudden and sharp rise in these disorders throughout Europe and the US over the past few decades (British Medical Journal News, 3rd June, 1995). In the UK this has been occurring within the context of a dramatic widening of the social inequality gap over the recent decades, with by far the biggest group affected being lower income families with children (Bradshaw, 1990).

As I discussed in Chapter 4, changes in social, political and economic circumstances have an effect on our cultural beliefs and value systems. This can result in changes in the meaning and significance we give to certain behaviours, the likelihood of certain behaviours occurring and how we go about the task of enlisting help to try and solve the problems we face.

In this context, parents, teachers, health professionals and other professionals right up to politicians, are looking for more explanations and ways of trying to cope and deal with these increasing difficulties, and are possibly looking for new scapegoats. In this culture the biomedical model has such cultural power that it is not unreasonable for most of the population to assume that once doctors have named certain behaviours as a disorder (which most people will interpret as medical illness), then this disorder must have a natural and scientific basis. The ADHD construct as a biomedical disorder has been ideally placed to respond to growing cultural anxieties (parental, professional and governmental) about children's development and well being, and it is well placed to give the illusion of addressing some of the painful and worrying social developments that have been taking place.

Within psychiatry, as discussed above, there are a number of competing explanations with much confusion about how to define and clarify the boundaries between ADHD and other externalizing disorders. Marked differences are observable between countries, within countries and between individual practitioners. As with other psychiatric categories, psychiatrists try to settle these disputes by developing a consensus (i.e. the most powerful and influential psychiatrists at any time decide how the borders of any category, and the category itself, should be defined) not by the development of any medically valid tests. The differences noted between the perceptions of medical professionals, however, still exist within a linear medical-model approach with (as regards to externalized behaviour in boys) two basic competing explanatory models being apparent. The first is that the problem is something to do with the parents, i.e. the parent-blame model. The second is that it's something to do with the child, i.e. the child-blame model. Where there is an issue of concern about blame and also where there is an issue of how difficult it is to do anything about these problems quickly, an interactive, more complex model is very difficult to sustain. In other words, both models have the price of distancing all concerned from the messy business of trying to understand the role of relationships, emotions and complex, wider, cultural factors.

But there are locally available western-culture-generated alternatives to the medical model for understanding ADHD-type behaviours. Let me consider a few alternative mental-health-culture-derived models.

> Perry and his co-workers (1995), pursuing a neuro biological approach, developed a hypothesis that follows from the above considerations. They started by noting how the symptoms of ADD/ADHD closely parallel those that occur during trauma – the hyper-alertness, the need to act quickly, the need to be on the qui vive at all times in the expectation of danger and the inability to turn attention to matters other than those of physical safety. Their hypothesis is that, in a critical period in infancy some children experience trauma, which initiates a habitual automatic response, as though to some external threat. When older such children are sensitive to threat to a much greater extent than other children are and revert, as it were, to a state of 'red alert' very easily. Thus as with post-traumatic stress, such children react quickly, over-actively, and not so much to their ordinary life as to anticipated threat. Perry, taking up an intergenerational position, is not concerned to blame parents for traumatising infants, but rather to point out that what is traumatic to an adult may not be traumatic to a child and vice versa.
>
> (Offord, 1998: 260)

The emphasis on internal psychological trauma is rather typical of a psycho-analytic-type explanation and belief system. Other psychodynamic ideas include hyperactivity as an attempt to ward off feelings of sadness and helplessness (Furman, 1974, 1996) and hyperactivity as a powerful communication from a child to get under the skin of an adult and let them know about the presence of very painful affects (Widener, 1998).

Moving outwards from internal-world explanatory models there are a variety of other models put forward as possible causes or explanations for ADHD-type behaviours. Breggin (1994, 1997) believes the absent father is, in most cases, an underlying cause of children's acting-out behaviour and has renamed ADD, DADD (Dad's attention deficit disorder). He believes that loving attention from their fathers is an effective curative factor for these children. Another theory relates to the effect an accumulation of stresses has on a family (e.g. lack of support, unresolved loss, poor relationship with father, insufficiently positive maternal model, pregnancy and birth complications, and difficult infant temperament). In such families, it is hypothesized, increasingly negative interactions develop between child and parent leading to exhaustion, frustration and irritability in the parent and challenging and hyperactive behaviour in the growing child, this in turn leads to a reinforcing demand–dissatisfaction cycle (Stiefel, 1997). Attachment theory is another popular framework amongst both family therapists and psychotherapists. Within an attachment framework, Lieberman and Pawl (1990), argue that impulsivity, recklessness, negative attention seeking, hyperactivity and poor concentration may represent a defensive adaptation on the part of a child in the context of an insecure attachment relationship. Similarly, Speltz (1990) interprets the dyscontrol and non-compliance of young insecurely attached children who use problem behaviour as an attempt to control the proximity of the caregiver.

Another aetiological model, this time based on a post-modern analysis of discourse and power, suggests that a mother-blaming culture may be an important factor in the rise of ADHD diagnoses. In this explanatory model, mothers who hear the negative judgements of school and other parents, experience a profound sense of self-blame, failure, guilt and helplessness, as well as anger and frustration at the child. When put in contact with the ADHD industry such a mother may, at least temporarily, feel freed from the mother-blaming context that has been so oppressive. She is no longer a failed mother, but a mother battling against the odds with a disabled child. In this analysis, the primary problem is not seen as residing in the mother or the child, but in the effects of the dominant discourses of psychology, psychiatry and patriarchy, which render parent and child as passive and separated from their abilities, competence and strengths (Law, 1997).

All the above mental-health models are meant to generate general hypotheses, which may or may not be relevant to particular children and families seen clinically. None, in my view, represents the discovery of an overarching, more powerful 'truth' (or core pathology) about ADHD-labelled children.

Moving out of mainstream mental-health cultures I've encountered many other potential explanations for ADHD-type behaviours from talking to colleagues, friends, relatives and, of course, the clients I work with. The explanations range from what I see as theories about changes in our cultural perceptions of what constitutes a problem (e.g. 'Boys used to be boys, but do some now see boyhood as a malady?' (Zachary, 1997)), often arguing that our culture has become child unfriendly and now discriminates against boys, to theories suggesting that there have been real changes in children's behaviours that are environmentally caused. When you keep your ear to the ground you soon realize that within our (and any other) current, everyday culture there are a large variety of rich, often complex explanations being thought about by a variety of people (particularly parents) who are trying to make some meaningful sense of the difficult task of bringing up children in a safe and positive way in this complicated day and age.

Here are a few of these explanations.

The pace of life has changed dramatically. We live in time-bound, competitive environments in which we have to always be on the go, always have a hundred and one things to achieve. Our daily living environments are full of sensory stimulation (visual, auditory, etc.) with time for doing nothing, meditating, reflecting on higher powers and your own insignificance, having been slowly squeezed to the margins of our culture. Independence, self-reliance and self-interest are the new gods, the new values ruling our lives and influencing us from a young age. In this cultural context, ADHD symptoms reflect the attempts of normal children and adults trying to adapt to these modern pressures and values. Attention deficit hyperactivity disorder is viewed as a problem in our children but it can aid adaptation to this frenetic world as an adult. Attention deficity hyperactivity disorder-type behaviours are thus an integral part of valued personality traits in modern culture and therefore encouraged by many media, but they are frowned upon in public spaces.

Another theory: children are not learning to control their impulses as they used to in the past. In the past, with parents having limited disposable income and there being fewer readily available sources of instant gratification, children had to learn through necessity to control their impulses. Nowadays, with instant gratification being such a big feature of the consumer culture, children are no longer being forced to learn early self-control of their impulses.

Another theory: children are being fed with hyperactive, often violent, role models such as power rangers and Pokemon. These characters are copied and identified with, particularly by boys, from very young vulnerable ages.

Another theory: life has become difficult for parents who are caught in a double pressure when it comes to discipline. On the one hand there are increased expectations for children to show restraint and self-control from an early age. On the other hand there is considerable social fear in parents generated by a culture of children's rights that often pathologizes normal, well-intentioned parents' attempts to discipline their children. Parents are left fearing a visit from the social services and the whole area of discipline becomes loaded with anxiety. This argument holds equally true for schools. Parents often criticize schools for lack of discipline. Schools often criticize parents for lack of discipline. This double bind has resulted in more power going to children who are too young to handle it and who are consequently more likely to go off the rails. For many children with ADHD the basic problem is a breakdown of their relationship to authority.

Another theory: we have become a child-unfriendly society. Children are potential consumers and are targeted by advertisers, professionals, etc. In such a culture children are increasingly being given the message that they are like adults. Parents are being given the message that their children are more like adults and should always be talked to, reasoned with, allowed to make choices, etc. An example of this that I can give relates to a visit to our health visitor when our son was just over a year old and we were expecting the birth of our daughter soon. The health visitor asked us if we had sat our son down and explained to him what was going to happen, otherwise he might become very jealous! In this culture, so the argument goes, kids can't be kids anymore, dependent, helpless, in need of rules, protection, values and authority, and there is nothing more likely to set a kid on the path to being out of control than giving him/her more power, responsibility and independence than they are developmentally capable of dealing with.

Another theory: there is a lack of common ownership of rules and values with regard to bringing up children, therefore children learn that only certain individuals have any right to make demands and have expectations with regard to their behaviour. Thus children can play adults off against each other more easily these days.

Another theory: junk diets, fizzy drinks, excessive consumption of crisps and chocolate, and the increasing amount of chemical additives in our children's diets is causing many behaviour problems, including hyperactivity and impulsiveness. This is because such diets lack vital nutrients as well as causing children to develop low-grade allergic reactions to the unnatural chemicals they contain.

Another theory: modern teaching methods result in too much emphasis on self-regulation and too little on clear structure and spoon feeding (dependency), resulting in a poor environment for children who have problems with organizing, ordering and learning and whose restlessness and poor concentration is subsequently intensified.

Another theory: classroom environments are over-stimulating, offer too much choice and therefore encourage distraction and poor concentration.

Another theory: children with poor self-esteem find that they can get a laugh (which for them is a form of temporary enjoyable attention and boost in self-esteem) by being the hyperactive class clown.

Another theory: in a culture with such high expectations of independence, self-reliance and responsibility, ADHD is one of the culturally acceptable ways of opting out. 'I can't help it, I have ADHD' can be used as an excuse for many things such as not doing homework, not enforcing discipline, the inability to hold down a relationship and so on.

Another theory: some are motivated by discovering that ADHD is a new convenient way of getting a label from which you can get extra disability benefits.

Another theory: children are like caged animals these days and their restlessness can be put down to the anxiety many parents have about their children's safety.

With reports of violence, kidnapping, drugs and other dangers, parents feel they have to keep their children indoors for their own safety.

Another theory: domestic violence can cause ADHD-type behaviours in some children by modelling impulsivity, aggression and disinhibition and by traumatizing children and putting them in a permanent state of being 'on the run'.

Another theory: some children develop ADHD behaviours as a direct result of chronic child abuse (physical, sexual and emotional abuse and neglect), or as a Munchausen's syndrome by proxy situation (where a parent needs their child to have a disorder for the purpose of getting attention themselves).

There are more theories that could be added to the above list and this is without even touching on the subject of explanatory models that may be encountered in non-western cultures. What I will say is that my experience of growing up in a non-western culture and of working with families from non-western backgrounds, leads me to agree with the suggestion of many that having the family, not the individual, as the primary social unit has a massive impact, not only on beliefs and values, but also directly on behaviour.

Hierarchy and power in attention deficit hyperactivity disorder

If you have followed my arguments so far I am suggesting that to best understand what ADHD is all about we have to look beyond the confines of the definition and consider the cultural context in which the ADHD construct has came about. Thus, so far I have followed the arguments I developed in Chapters 3 and 4, namely, that to believe in ADHD requires an act of faith on the part of the believer in the construct that ADHD is one of many models that can be used to explain and understand these types of behaviour. In this section I am going to suggest that the reason why ADHD has become so popular as an explanation at this moment in time is best understood by examining the issue of hierarchy and power.

Attention deficit hyperactivity disorder is a popular and popularized construct because it comes from the medical profession which continues to have a high status in this culture. The belief amongst those scientific priests of ADHD, is that it is a discoverable condition on which we can build scientific knowledge, even though they have started building the institute without first building the foundations. A jump in logic has taken place. Basically, some observable behaviours in children (such as inattention and hyperactivity) have changed in status from being behaviours that contain no more or less information (in isolation) than the inattention or hyperactivity as described by an observer, to becoming the basis of a primary diagnosis. The biomedical template is applied and the behaviours are interpreted as a disorder. This leaves out several layers of experience and context that could contribute to any observed behaviour as well as the meaning given to the behaviour. This medical, explanatory model has enormous cultural power. Naturally, most of the population will assume that once doctors have named these behaviours as a disorder, such a categorization must have a natural, scientific basis.

This diagnostic label then gives the impression that children with the label are similar and minimizes their many differences. Once the cultural idea of the ADHD construct becomes rooted in everyday culture, children experiencing difficulties caused by a variety of complex processes can now be given the label of an illness, such a label then creates the illusion that information, advice and scientific understanding of the child's condition is now available.

As I argued above, anxieties about children's development and behaviour has grown enormously in modern, western societies in recent times. In the hierarchy of professional relationships, medicine is in a strong position to influence the other professions that are also trying to deal with this growing anxiety about children. In the US and Canada, behavioural psychologists, trusting that neurologists would, in time, discover the characteristics of the central nervous system that makes behavioural categorizations valid (Homans, 1993), took up the disorder and along with medical institutions passed the concept on to educationalists and eventually policy makers (US Department of Education, 1991). Thus, the medical profession has been ideally placed to influence other professions and eventually government policy, leading to the popularization of the concept and ever widening boundaries of its definition. Once there has been greater cultural popularization of this idea, children (particularly boys) who are either failing academically or exhibiting behavioural problems at home or at school are suspected by a wide variety of professionals, parents, relatives and other influential people in the child's life, of having ADHD. The highly subjective nature of the DSM-IV definition allows for some very liberal interpretations, making ADHD well placed as a potential dumping ground for a whole host of problems. Wolraich *et al.* (1990) showed that in only 30 per cent of already diagnosed children in their study, did the home and school report both fulfil the DSM diagnostic criteria.

In addition to the ADHD construct being in an ideal position to act as a cultural defence mechanism, its popularity has been further strengthened through the growing interests in the merits of prescribing stimulant medication to children. There is little doubt that in the short term methylphenidate hydrochloride, commonly known as Ritalin®, (the stimulant most frequently prescribed to children) results in clinical improvement in many children who show hyperactivity and poor attention, with decreases in motor activity and defiance frequently reported (Schachar and Tannock, 1997, Greenhill, 1998). This observation has acted as a powerful reinforcer of the ADHD construct, many interpreting this as confirmatory evidence of the suspected physical causation (and therefore treatment) of the disorder. However, the evidence suggests that the effects of stimulants on the central nervous system are not limited to those children who can be defined by the boundaries of this disorder. Thus stimulants have been found to have the same cognitive and behavioural effects on otherwise normal children (Rapoport *et al.*, 1978, 1980; Donnelly and Rapoport, 1985; Garber *et al.*, 1996; Zahn *et al.*, 1980), aggressive children regardless of diagnosis (Campbell *et al.*, 1982; Spencer *et al.*, 1996) and children with comorbid conduct disorder (Taylor *et al.*, 1987; Spencer *et al.*, 1996). This is not surprising. The pharmacological action of Ritalin® on the brain is basically that of amphetamines (or 'speed', its street name) and cocaine (Volkow *et al.*, 1995). Adults who abuse drugs such as speed get a high, one of whose components is a capacity to hyper-focus into very particular and intensely experienced sensory inputs (for example music). This psychochemical effect occurs in most, but not all, of those who take speed. Similarly, when given to children, this psychochemical effect is not diagnosis dependent.

Research has focused almost exclusively on short-term outcomes. Why so few long-term studies from the manufacturers? Huynh *et al.* (1999), in their medium-term outcome study, discovered that between 30 and 50 per cent of children treated for an average of 64 weeks on Ritalin® had a poor outcome. This was particularly so for the group receiving significantly higher doses of the stimulant medication. This fits with my, and many of my colleague's, clinical experience of children becoming tolerant to increasing doses of Ritalin®. The few long-term studies which have been conducted suggest that stimulants do not result in any long-term improvement in either behavioural or academic achievement (Weis *et al.*, 1975; Rie *et al.*, 1976; Charles and Schain, 1981; Gadow, 1983; Hetchman *et al.*, 1984; Klein and Mannuzza, 1991). This concurs with the clinical impression that a lot can be gained from a cautious approach to prescribing Ritalin® and treating it as a window of opportunity, and little by treating it as a wonder drug. Despite the complete lack of evidence for any long-term effectiveness, Ritalin® is most usually prescribed continuously for 7, 8 or more years, with children as young as 3 years old being prescribed the drug, despite the manufacturer's licence stating that it should not be prescribed to children under 6 years (Baldwin and Cooper, 2000).

Outcome research in Ritalin® treatment has been shown to have serious short-falls in methodology, such as the use of small samples, inadequate description of randomization or blinding, and not accounting for withdrawals or drop outs (Zwi *et al.*, 2000). Most recently a big fuss has been made about a large multi-centre trial in the US, testing the efficacy of Ritalin® (MTA Co-operative Group, 1999a, 1999b). I recently heard an eminent professor of child psychiatry in the UK state, at a large conference attended by child psychiatrists and paediatricians, that the implication of the results of this study is that we should be treating children with ADHD with medication as the first-line treatment and possibly without any other intervention. This extraordinarily narrow interpretation of the results shows how some clinicians are hell bent on stripping all context and controversy to bolster their beliefs, without regard for the enormous impact such statements may have on clinical practice in this country.

The study in question compared four groups of children who were given one of four treatments: medication only, intensive behavioural treatment, combined behavioural treatment and medication, or standard community care. The study concluded that the medication-only and combined behavioural and medication groups had the best outcome, with the combined group having only a marginally better outcome than the medication-only group. A closer look inevitably brings up important questions of how to interpret the significance of these results. As with other studies, serious methodological issues have been pointed out in relation to this one (Boyle and Jadad, 1999). The findings are not particularly remarkable and even at face value only confirm what we already know, namely that this powerful medication has the potential to bring about large changes in behaviour in the short term (this study lasted 14 months, a long way off the many years Ritalin® is usually prescribed). The comparison psychological treatment of behaviour therapy is another approach based on a medical linear construct and therefore of questionable quality. Presumably all those (researchers and their subjects) in the study are assuming there is such a 'biological' thing as ADHD and so are already being cultured into a disability mode. Many of the behaviour therapies were given by medical staff not trained in behaviour therapy (Breggin, 2000). Then there's the small print, the bits that aren't noticed if you only advertise the particular bias of the conclusion. All four groups in the treatment programme showed sizable reductions in symptoms. The conclusion could have read 'children not on medication made enormous improvements'. The conclusion that medication only is perhaps the best treatment for ADHD, reflects the interests and agenda of the researchers who were most interested in rating ADHD-type behaviours, not necessarily those of the parents or their children. Two thirds of the community-treated group were also receiving stimulant medication during the period of the study, yet were placed in the poorer outcome category. Many of the researchers were funded by the drug industry. Of course it is in the drug companies' interests to highlight studies and conclusions that are likely to enhance their products sales, after all who knows how many negative trials whose results don't please the drug companies have been discarded by them (Ruesch, 1992). Where there is a conflict between giving accurate information and making sales it is not always the worthier motive that carries the day.

The dogma from ADHD priests stating that Ritalin® is a safe drug with few harmful side effects couldn't be further from the truth. Troublesome and frequently reported side effects include poor appetite, weight loss, growth suppression, insomnia, depression, irritability, confusion and mood swings, a flattening of the emotions giving the individual a zombie-like appearance, stomach ache, headaches, staring, disinterest, tachycardia, pituitary dysfunction and dizziness (Barkley *et al.*, 1990; Breggin, 1999). Cramond (1994) has also reported that treatment with Ritalin® is associated with lowered self-esteem and suppression of creativity in some children. Ritalin® may also have long-term adverse effects in as many as one third of those treated, including subtle cognitive effects such as perseveration, preoccupations, sombreness and deterioration in performance on complex cognitive tasks (Solanto and Wender, 1989; Sprague and Sleator, 1977). The lack of long-term studies into the effects of Ritalin® and other stimulants is a concern as we do not really know what sort of effect an amphetamine-like substance has on the developing brain. This is particularly so, as psychostimulants are powerful amphetamine-like drugs with potentially addictive properties. Children become tolerant to the effects of psychostimulants and are given gradually increasing doses as the years on a drug clock up. The potential for tolerance and addiction is further demonstrated by withdrawal states (known as the rebound effect which manifests in increased excitability, activity, talkativeness, irritability and insomnia) seen when the last dose of the day is wearing off or when the drug is withdrawn suddenly (Barkley *et al.*, 1990; Breggin, 1998).

More difficult to assess is the possible socio-cultural effects that such widespread use of stimulants in children may have. Doctors may be unwittingly convincing children to control and manage themselves using medication, a pattern that may carry on into adulthood as the preferred or only way to cope with life's stresses. Clinically I often come across children on stimulants that have admitted that they were secretly self-medicating at times of stress. Parents, teachers and others may lose interest in understanding the meaning behind an ADHD-labelled child's behaviour, beyond that of an illness internal to the child that needs medication. Variation in the diagnosis and treatment between different social classes in the US and Canada, with ADHD being diagnosed far more frequently amongst children from families of low socio-economic status, has led some authors to conclude that Ritalin® is being misused as a drug for social control of children from disadvantaged communities (McGuinness, 1989; Kohn, 1989). The National Association for the Advancement of Colored People in the US has offered strong testimony that young blacks are over-represented in the ADHD category and are over-medicated, and it has been campaigning for black parents to reject such a diagnosis (British Psychological Society, 1996). In the UK the parent support group, 'Overload', has been campaigning for prescribing doctors to provide more information to parents about the cardiovascular and neurological side effects of psychostimulants, believing that many more parents would be likely to reject such medication if they were properly informed about it by the medical profession.

Ritalin® has recently emerged as a new drug of abuse as it can be crushed and snorted to produce a high (Heyman, 1994). Surveys have shown that a significant proportion of adolescents in the US self-report using Ritalin® for non-medical purposes (Robin and Barkley, 1998). The neurochemical effects of Ritalin® are very similar to that of cocaine, which is one of the most addictive drugs known. Cocaine users report that the effect of injected Ritalin® is almost indistinguishable from that of cocaine (Volkow *et al.*, 1995) and the jury is still out as to whether using Ritalin® will increase, decrease, or have no effect on the chances of drug abuse later in life. In Italy the Ministry of Health banned the prescription of stimulants, including methylphenidate, following concerns about its potential for misuse (Gallucci *et al.*, 1993). Ritalin® remains a controversial drug for reasons that go well beyond its side effects. Yet these issues that should be important information for all parents trying to make the difficult decision as to whether or not to agree for their children to be prescribed a stimulant, is information that is rarely given by the prescribers (Baldwin and Cooper, 2000).

Despite these contradictions and concerns the availability of a drug that is believed to treat a childhood biomedical illness has proved so attractive that prescription levels, certainly in the US and Canada and more recently in the UK, have spiralled to reach what some consider to be epidemic proportions. General practitioners and paediatricians as well as child psychiatrists routinely prescribe stimulants to children in the US and Canada. National surveys of paediatricians (Copeland *et al.*, 1987) and family practitioners (Wolraich *et al.*, 1990) in the US have found that over 80 per cent of children diagnosed as having ADHD were treated with Ritalin®. National consumption of Ritalin® in the US more than doubled between 1981 and 1992 (Drug Enforcement Administration, 1994) with surveys estimating that in the late 1980s as many as 6 per cent of American public elementary school children were receiving stimulants (Safer and Kraeger, 1988). Prescriptions of Ritalin® have continued to increase in the 1990s, with one source quoting that over 11 million prescriptions of Ritalin® had been written in 1996 in the US (McGinnis, 1997). One shocking 1995 state survey of teachers found that nearly 40 per cent of elementary school and 32 per cent of junior high students were diagnosed as having ADHD and medicated with stimulants (Runnheim, 1996). Of the children placed on psychostimulants, 80 to 90 per cent are boys (Zachary, 1997).

This phenomenal rise in the use of psychostimulants has led to the suggestion that ADHD has been conceived and promoted by the pharmaceutical industry in order for there to be an entity for which stimulants could be prescribed (McGuinness, 1989). It is, after all, a multi-million-dollar industry, with the National Institute of Mental Health (Karon, 1994), the US Department of Education (Merrow, 1995) and the Food and Drug Administration (Breggin, 1994, 1997) all having been involved in funding and promoting the medication of children with behavioural problems. In the US the manufacturers of Ritalin® now face legal action alleging that they are responsible for fraud and conspiracy. It is claimed that the pharmaceutical companies Ciba & Novartis conspired and colluded to develop and promote the diagnosis of ADHD in a highly successful effort to increase the market for its product, Ritalin®. This effort has included funding parent support groups as well as outcome research and payments to professionals (Waters and Kraus, 2000).

The cultural preconditions for ADHD to become a popular concept have come about in the UK as they did in the US. In response to the current cultural anxieties the types of solutions attempted are, by and large, culture specific. In this culture it means a market place commodity or consumer-driven solution. Anyone who works in the health service in the UK these days, knows how much the culture in the health service has shifted towards a management-driven culture with management 'speak' being evident in the decision-making bodies. This in turn leads to a way in which the practice of medicine itself is influenced by issues of the hierarchy and power in the wider culture. In a health service becoming dominated by market-driven thinking (which has obviously influenced the private sector for a long time) service developments have to adapt their thinking to fit into this powerful influence on its own development.

Attention deficiency hyperactivity disorder has recently received a lot of coverage in the popular media in the UK. Most articles and programmes have advocated using this label (explicitly and implicitly by referring to ADHD and not, for example, hyperkinetic syndrome), often citing examples of medical practice in the US and Canada for comparison (although some newspaper articles have occasionally raised concerns, they have tended to be in the middle-class-read broadsheets). Pressure groups such as LADDER and ADDIS have, understandably, taken up ADHD as a medical concept and have become increasingly vocal in advocating the use of the American DSM label ADHD and the prescription of stimulant medication. In the US and Canada the national parent support group, Children and Adults with Attention Deficit Disorder (CHADD) has become a very powerful body defining ADHD as a 'neurobiological thing'. CHADD, not surprisingly, receives significant funding from the drug company that makes Ritalin® (Merrow, 1995). The process of the powerful medical establishment passing on the idea of there being a discoverable, biological disorder to the public, having taken place, the effects of the consequent consumer pressure is already showing. Demand from parents, teachers, educational psychologists and general practitioners for ADHD assessments and for consideration of the prescription of stimulants, has increased enormously in the past few years with the consequent development of specialist private and National Health Service ADHD clinics in the UK.

The notion of ADHD is seductive and influential on practitioners as well as consumers. The encounter of doctor and patient follows a well-known cultural script involving a dependent sufferer and a healthy expert who is assumed to possess the skills and knowledge to diagnose an illness, have information about that illness and provide a treatment. In child psychiatry practitioners have had to largely work outside this script in attempting to engage with the ambiguities and anxieties that children, their families and other professionals bring, a process that can be slow and stressful for the practitioner as well as their clients. Attention deficit hyperactivity disorder is perhaps the first childhood psychiatric disorder where the traditional cultural script for doctor and patient can be followed. It thus has the potential to be packaged and marketed as a commodity. As Freud noted, all cultures struggle with the difficult question of how to gain control over that source of suffering that comes from interpersonal relationships, and all cultures develop ways of trying to regulate this complex area of life in an effort to try to reduce the suffering and the negative emotion that comes with it (see Chapter 4). In this sense I believe that ADHD can be seen as one of the most recent cultural defence mechanisms that has been generated and invented as a cultural way of trying to deal with the growing anxieties about childhood development that are clearly present in modern, western culture. In such a scenario where no real expert knowledge on ADHD can be said to exist, the wish to define this disorder becomes complicit with clients' and families' wishes to be controlled, to feel that there is certainty, an answer where really there is only uncertainty and questions.

A multi-perspective approach

So far in this chapter I have examined the concept of ADHD in accordance with the analysis I used in Chapters 3, 4 and 5 of this book. I have concluded that ADHD is a concept that depends more on the faith of the practitioner than on any scientific evidence, that ADHD is one of many possible conceptual frameworks that can be used to shed light on children with these behaviours, and that ADHD's current popularity has much to do with the dynamics of power and hierarchy. In this section I will put forward an alternative model for working with children who could be diagnosed as having ADHD and with their families. This model was used in an ADHD service in London that I was involved in setting up. The clinic was set up with the idea of trying to incorporate wider contextual issues and developing more multi-perspective interventions.

It's difficult in a few lines to give a full and rich account of using this approach in clinical practice with children referred for ADHD assessments, as each member of staff in a clinic brings their own character, beliefs and perspectives into the melting pot. It's important from the outset that these multiple perspectives are valued, listened to and worked with despite the inevitable disagreements that will happen. Staff, like clients I believe, need to be able to feel that they are respected and valued and can think and act relatively freely if they are going to be able to be themselves, and feel motivated and effective, when working with their clients.

Before talking about the guidelines we used in helping us structure our clinical work in this clinic, I would like to mention the actual title of the clinic. We decided to call the clinic 'The clinic for ADHD and other difficult to manage behaviours'. We had to include 'ADHD' in the title as the setting up of an ADHD clinic was the basis on which funding for the clinic was agreed. However, we were uncomfortable with simply calling it an ADHD clinic as we did not wish the primary role of this clinic to be a 'yes, you have it' or 'no, you don't' type of operation. Given the existing disagreements within professional circles, let alone non-professional ones, about what constitutes ADHD, we did not want the diagnosis to become a privilege which gave certain children and families a ticket to a service, and excluded others who may not reach a certain threshold but whose problems may mean they are in just as great a need of (and could benefit just as much from) the type of multi-disciplinary service this clinic would provide. Hence, for these political reasons we included in the title the phrase 'and other difficult to manage behaviours', to make it possible to continue working, where necessary, with those who had been referred to the clinic even if they had not been diagnosed as having ADHD.

The following is a summary of a few of the principles we have tried to adopt in running this clinic.

1. Slow down the assessment process and engage the system   We devised a three-stage approach to the assessment. The first appointment is clinic-based and is a first opportunity to meet the family and the child. At this meeting we try and gather some information and get some understanding of the family's stories. It is also the first opportunity to try and engage the child, find out their viewpoint and what (if anything) they would like to see change. The second stage, with the family's permission, is to make a school visit. Here we observe the child for half an hour in their classroom and then speak, usually, to the class teacher and/or the special-needs coordinator at the school. This gives us the opportunity to observe the child in their school and get some understanding of how the child is functioning in their school environment. For many children referred, school is the big issue for the parents. The third stage of the assessment is to make a home visit where we have another opportunity to observe the child in a different context and we also have the opportunity to meet the family on their territory. At this meeting we have an opportunity to feed back from our school meeting, make further observations of the child in a different context, develop our relationship with the child and their family, and gather further information. Finally, we have an appointment back at the clinic to complete the assessment, in which feedback, about our opinion so far, is given to the family. From the first appointment we show an interest in the family's and the child's ideas and beliefs. We are attempting to collect different stories about the child, in particular different explanations to account for the child's behaviour that different people or the same person puts forward. Throughout the assessment we are using our clinical judgement to approach sessions flexibly. Frequently opportunities for what might be considered treatment arise during the assessment, thus we also view the assessment period as the first opportunity to begin interventions. Sometimes just the whole process of bringing different bits of the system together can, in itself, make all the difference needed. We are also trying to slow down the process so that from the start we are introducing the idea that our job is not to simply focus on a 'yes he has it' or 'no he doesn't' medical test kind of approach.

2. Put a lot of effort into trying to engage children and their families   Many families who come to the clinic have had previous referrals to child and adolescent mental-health services and other agencies (perhaps social services, education psychology, educational welfare, private clinics, etc.). They sometimes have a history of repeated referrals and frequent failures to attend. This may reflect the nature of how some families feel about helping agencies, possibly experiencing them as blaming or perhaps even fearing that these agencies may take their children away. With many of these difficult-to-engage clients, a patient, long-term approach is needed. Making home visits and school visits may help these clients to feel more respected and understood, particularly if they feel you're making an effort to get out of your office to see their child in different situations and meet them on their own territory. There's a lot that can be done to make it possible for clients who have had difficult relationships with helping agencies to develop a different feeling about that helping agency (and maybe other helping agencies). For example, steering clear of any suggestions on how to parent may be important. Suggestions on how to parent can be experienced as blaming and undermining, and are not welcome from someone who knows little about that family and how they bring up their children. Instead picking up on any cues you find of examples of good parenting, or clear examples of how dedicated the parents appear to be towards their children, can be experienced as positive and trust building. Obviously there are important precautions to be taken as you don't want to be condoning abusive situations. In my experience, however, the vast majority of these difficult-to-engage clients are not abusive to their children but, perhaps because of class or cultural issues, their style of parenting and the way they express their love for their children and their dedication to their children may have been misinterpreted as abuse by the predominantly white middle-class agencies (e.g. teachers, psychologists, social services). Even if such a thing had not happened, the parents themselves may fear it will happen. There are other simple things that can be done to help the parents feel that you're on their side, such as letters to housing, social services, supporting a recommendation for statementing and so on. Children too may come in a suspicious, defensive frame of mind, fearing more telling off and blame. I try to look for the positives in any account and show much more curiosity and interest in these aspects. I often focus questions and comments a lot more around the functional, coping and thoughtful aspects of the child. If a child is completely hostile, then a more playful approach can be rewarding, for example give them easy challenges and tell them that you bet they can't do it and express surprise when they do.

3. Take a multifactorial approach   That is try to move families from single-explanation approaches (ADHD is often approached as if it is an explanation whereas, as I have mentioned above, it is only a description of behaviour) to including all other explanations available. These may come up through our own opinions during the assessment but often are explanations that families, schools and others have put forward, but whose significance has been pushed down in status as being less meaningful than ADHD as an explanation. Thus, clinically, we try during the assessment and afterwards to continually rehabilitate complexity. The alternative explanations that are often put forward, which seem to me just as valid if not more so as ADHD is not an explanation *per se*, include things such as learning difficulties with consequent low threshold of frustration and low self confidence, a child full of energy who is not getting enough exercise, an emotionally troubled child who will not express himself (e.g. no longer having contact with their father, witnessed domestic violence, a victim of bullying, etc.), a child using his intelligence to work out how to get round people, a child having a problem with his temper or not getting enough sleep, a child finding the only way he can get attention is to be the class clown, a child that likes being hyperactive, is copying his father or has no respect for authority, and so on. It's very easy to miss these everyday explanations that many parents and children have about why they are the way they are and it's very easy to give these explanations no significance at all. Once you look out for these simple, everyday explanations they can be found, and have been found in every case that I have come across so far. Many of these explanations exist but need to be actively searched for as they are relegated to a lower status than the assumed possibility of ADHD, particularly if the family is meeting a doctor from an ADHD clinic! This does not mean that the illness model isn't a useful one (particularly in the early stages), but to keep trying to open this model up and to keep thinking alive may be more important.

4. Take a slow-process approach to deconstructing the meaning behind a diagnosis of ADHD I try to be open with clients about the controversies relating to ADHD in a fairly straightforward manner. For example, I might explain quite early on that there is no such thing as a test for ADHD and in that sense it's different to diagnoses such as pneumonia or diabetes where you can take a blood sample or an x-ray, in other words do actual tests to help substantiate the diagnosis. I explain that the diagnosis is based on clinical judgement and explain about the types of behaviours we look for in making the diagnosis. I also explain that there is disagreement, both historically and currently, about how to arrive at the diagnosis, with different countries and different clinicians having different ideas about the cut off between normal and disorder. I explain that the cause is unknown with different clinicians having different opinions about what might cause it and whether it needs to be present at home, at school and everywhere else or just in one place. The aim of taking this approach is to get the idea across that the ADHD label does not provide an explanation, it does not answer the 'why' question, at least not in our current state of knowledge. I try to do this to reduce the potential of ADHD being over-used as an explanation which then closes down the possibilities for looking at other potentially useful avenues for explaining and trying to understand a child's behaviour. If the meaning behind an ADHD diagnosis is not opened up you can get that dreadful equation that sometimes arises in those who have been too vigorously cultured into the ADHD faith of, when a problem arises with a child who has a diagnosis of ADHD, the first question on the lips of the faithful (be they the parents, teachers or even the child themselves) is 'what's happening with the medication?' ('has he taken it?' 'does he need more?'). This is a very understandable reaction but, from my clinical experience, seems to lead to a rather disastrous, no-win situation, where the only way to deal with problems becomes that of increasing medication. As a result, a number of the more religious clinicians have found themselves going well beyond the licensed maximum dose for Ritalin® (I often hear of adolescents who are on two to three times the maximum licensed dose for Ritalin®. To me this is no different than the medical profession creating a drug addict). Other religious practitioners have found themselves introducing other, untested medications in addition to Ritalin®, such as risperidone which is a powerful anti-psychotic drug with the potential for those on long-term treatment with this drug to have a permanent, untreatable movement disorder. This does not mean we should not discuss with the family and the child, whether this child does meet the criteria for ADHD and indeed which criteria they might meet. It is also important to know that for many families having the diagnosis may be helpful in the first instance as they may feel that they have an explanation, a way forward, some hope that things can begin to change and something to tell other people. Furthermore, they may feel that at last others, and not just them as parents, have recognized that their child has a problem. So sometimes it is helpful for families to go through the process of diagnosis at the same time as beginning the process of deconstructing its meaning and maintaining all the other explanations that may be helpful to pursue (including those related to the parents' style of parenting).

5. Look for the positives and for solutions the family have already generated
When families come to the clinic they are clearly there because of problems they or someone else (e.g. the school) is having with the child. Thus the session(s) will be dominated by problem talk usually in front of the child concerned. Of course it's important to listen carefully and try to understand the nature of the difficulties the child, family and others are experiencing. However, I often make an active attempt right from the first session to look for the positives and/or descriptions of the child that don't fit with the dominant story being given. For example, towards the end of the first session I may say something like 'I know that the reason you've come here today is because of all the problems you're having with Andy and you've given me a lot of useful information about all of that. But you know I'm also very interested in finding out about what's good about Andy and what's been going well or just better with him. It'll help me understand some of Andy's other sides to himself if you know what I mean.' It's not unusual for families to take a while before they can adjust their frame of mind to start talking about these aspects and often I have to persist. I do that by saying things like 'I know what you're saying, that nothing is going well and nothing has improved and of course that's why you came here to get help with these problems, but I still find it worth it, to just find out about some things, however small, however insignificant where there wasn't a problem or where things went well even if it was just for a few minutes, it'll just give me a fuller picture of what else is going on with Andy.' Sometimes I open it up to anyone in the room, particularly the child themselves to come up with examples. Sometimes I focus it down 'Let's just take yesterday then, tell me something however short lived or small that was okay, for example he took a cup back to the kitchen, he kissed you good night, he spoke to his sister nicely, he got into school on time, anything, anything at all.' I have yet to come across a family who, given a bit of space, time and a touch of persistence on my part, hasn't come up with something. Furthermore, once they start it's nearly always the case that you get a list of at least five things, often more, that are okay or good (and that don't fit the dominant problem story). I often do this type of thing again in later sessions and refer back to the original list to compare how their child is now and see what has changed. Keeping hold of the big picture is, I believe, very important. For example 6 months or a year after you first started seeing a family, you may be bogged down in a rather hopeless feeling session where the family are telling you about a particular incident or difficulty they are currently trying to deal with in relation to their child. Yet overall you know the child has made significant progress. At a convenient moment you may try and bring this bigger picture into the session by asking a question like 'I know you're going through a tough time right now and are very worried about Andy, but can I just ask you to take a step back for a minute. For example can you remember what things were like when we first met about 10 months ago?' Then I go through a process of talking about what has or hasn't changed overall and how every recovery has setbacks (i.e. what you're going through is normal) and how often if you're in the middle of a setback the greatest fear is that you're going back to square one (but clearly Andy is not), etc. Keeping

the good news alive is important in all cases, but is particularly so where there seems to be a history of major attachment-type issues (in other words a lot of built-up hostility and negative feeling between a parent and child). Noticing solutions and amplifying them can also be of great benefit. By paying attention to a time, however small or seemingly insignificant, when the child wasn't all over the place and out of control, and getting everyone to think about what might have been different about this time (what was the child doing, what were the parents doing, what else was going on, etc.), you can begin to help parents and children rediscover their own competence and expertise. I often make a special effort at showing surprise at these moments when coping or solution stories emerge, 'hang on a minute run that past me again', 'really? Is that really what happened?', 'wow, that's amazing how did you manage that'. I often come back to these solution stories during a session in the hope that at least one participant might have experienced at least one part of the session as a time when they showed me what they are capable of, as opposed to what's wrong with them.

6. Be open and informative and allow the parents to make the decision about medication
I see my main duty where the use of medication is being considered, whether it's an issue that has been raised by myself, by another professional or by the parent(s), is to provide adequate information to allow the parent(s) to make an informed decision. This is particularly so for psychostimulants like Ritalin®, which after all is a controlled drug (prescriptions for controlled drugs have much stricter guidelines than non-controlled drugs, controlled drugs tend to be those drugs with a potential for being abused). Providing information means telling the clients about how the drug works, the evidence for its effectiveness, the side-effect profile and the types of controversies there are (both sides of the argument should be mentioned). For me, it also means telling clients what is factual (e.g. the side-effect profile) and what is my opinion. I am frequently asked for my advice on matters such as dosage and what type of regime should be used. I usually say something like 'well, this is my opinion on what I believe works best'. I explain that other doctors may well have very different opinions about this medication. My advice with psychostimulants, like Ritalin®, tends to be to keep the dose as low as possible for as long as possible, 4 pm should be the latest time in the day to take a tablet because of sleep interference problems if taken later, and to have at least 1 preferably 2 days a week without medication to minimize problems with tolerance and dependence, and to keep everyone searching and thinking about alternatives to medication so that they remain able to cope when their child is not taking it. I also encourage families to be flexible and creative in their use of medication. For example, many families can cope quite well during weekends and school holidays with their child not taking medication. However, when going out the child and family may experience problems and this may be the very thing that they feel the child and themselves need to do more of, in which case a tablet before they go out can be very helpful. This approach to medication also includes the idea that medication is not diagnosis dependent. Most parents can work very effectively with the idea that their child is benefiting from

medication even without the diagnosis. Many parents are enormously helped by the attitude that medication is a window of opportunity, not a cure and from the outset develop the idea that medication is being used to allow a breathing space for everyone to help the child achieve, maybe improve their self-confidence, gain friends and so on. Most parents seem to understand my approach and, I believe, are happy to be treated as the expert best placed to make decisions about their child. In my experience, most parents would like to avoid their child having to take medication if at all possible, and if their child is on medication they would like to see them come off it as soon as is practical. The providing of information, clarity about when an opinion is just an opinion, and giving the parents the choice and final say about medication is, I believe, an important part of helping parents feel that what is happening belongs to them and is under their control.

7. Be prepared to be in there for the long haul   Be patient – time often brings unexpected coincidences and new things to explore in a natural, unforced manner. There have been many times where certain coincidences or events, perhaps during a home visit, have opened up another layer of understanding to explore. I now feel less inclined to jump into theorizing and trying to find out too much information about a family (particularly things like the parents' own histories) until opportunities naturally present themselves and when there is a reasonable sense of trust established between myself and the family. Then I can start being more openly challenging and curious if necessary. Opportunities for looking at new explanations and new solutions frequently happen by chance. I've often gone on a home visit and there's been a friend of the family or a relative who has joined the conversation and either been open about an issue which I hadn't previously been made aware of by the family (e.g. 'he behaves like that because he knows if he makes a big enough fuss you'll give in to him') or has provided an alternative idea or description that opened new areas to explore. In one session I was told about a video of a documentary that a referred child's father had been in when he was about the same age as his child. The father then showed me clips of this video, which was essentially about the racism and cultural adjustment problems that second generation West Indian immigrant children were facing in British schools. The documentary used this father's families' story as its main focus. Watching this video with the father led to a lot of useful and informative discussions about the father's experiences and his beliefs, and generated quite a few alternative ideas and explanations with regard to his son's problems.

8. Be prepared to consider alternative approaches   Diet is frequently an issue that is brought up by parents. After starting this clinic we realized that diet and allergies and their relationship to children's behaviour was a topic we knew very little about. The topic was being brought up by parents and sometimes other professionals. We were open about the fact that we were at the bottom of the learning curve on this topic. Where parents are interested, we have given them any information we have had available (including leaflets on food supplements). Some parents have tried their children on the supplement 'Effalex' (a fish-oil-based supplement, claimed by the manufacturer to help some children with ADHD) and have reported significant improvements in their children after a few weeks on it. Some have wished to try exclusion diets. Generally our advice has been that where parents are interested in diet we have advised the sort of healthy diet that would be good for most children and that is as low in artificial chemicals as possible (this pretty much excludes junk foods, sweets, crisps, fizzy drinks, most tinned food and most meats).

9. Challenge and deconstruct the hierarchy   Give greater importance to the client's own knowledge and less importance to our own. Local knowledge is searched for and opened up and explored wherever possible. Attention deficit hyperactivity disorder would, in this context, be an example of professional knowledge, given that it's a concept created by professionals and requiring so-called specialist expertise to diagnose. The equivalent examples of local knowledge maybe something like 'he's just like his father'. This belief can be opened up and looked at further by asking certain questions. What are the sorts of things that he does that reminds you of his father? What sorts of things are not like his father? Who else does he remind you of sometimes? What sort of things do you think he has inherited from his father (and his mother)? In what sort of things do you think he copies his father (and his mother)? Does he look up to his dad?, etc. Common sense, grandparent, old-school-type advice is important to pick up on and follow through. Ideals, like children require nurturing, firm discipline, plenty of exercise, plenty of time to play, plenty of fresh air, good diet, routine and good sleep, have been known for hundreds of generations. This common sense everyday knowledge will always be relevant. As far as professional knowledge is concerned this is provided in an open non-prescriptive and non-top-down sort of manner. One obvious example is parenting. Professionals all too often act as if there is only one way to parent and any other way is harmful. The current convention in professional circles, is for a white middle-class style of parenting as enshrined in the cognitive behavioural, learning theory approach. I have no particular problems with this version of how to parent, indeed, like most mental-health professionals, I often use some of the principles in my own practice. What I believe is important, however, is to consider how this fits in with things like the practical reality for families (it seems to me cognitive behavioural therapy for behavioural problems in children has been designed for reasonably well-off families who have no more than two children), the nature of the family's relationship to the institution (or the institutional transference if you prefer that concept) and how it fits in with the family's own style of parenting (it seems to me that cognitive behavioural therapy works less well in families with strong emotional and physical closeness, like many families from an Indian sub-continent background). In working with families on parenting issues it's quite frequent to pick up in the conversation a principle from a behavioural intervention. If I do I move in quickly to make sure the family or individual own that bit of knowledge, for example by saying 'are you sure you didn't write the books that I learnt from? 'cos this is exactly what the psychology books say'. I might try and elaborate from there and say in the form of information some other things that are said in these psychology books. Sometimes I feel very strongly that a certain principle from theory needs to be put across (e.g. that a cycle of negative reinforcement is taking place), in which case I will explain this (i.e. explain that I feel a negative cycle is taking place and we must try to break this). At this point, if we are in agreement, I would ask for their ideas and tell them what the books say and perhaps something from my own experience both as a parent and as someone who has worked with other families who have had problems with their children. I have virtually stopped using standard behavioural diaries as it seems to put too many people off. Those who aren't put off often don't fill them in properly or honestly, and those who do fill them in properly and honestly seem to be the easy to engage group who respond to far simpler and shorter interventions. Another important aspect of deconstructing the hierarchy is, I believe, that of deconstructing the whole professional identity business. These days I feel I am a similar person at home and at work. I engage in a lot of chit-chat and small talk with clients. If anyone (client or other professional) wants me to call them by their first name, then I insist they call me by my first name. Given that I spend so much time prying into people's personal business, if someone asks me a personal question I will answer it honestly.

10. Transparency   I try not to keep ideas secret. If I have an idea then I share it, however difficult it might be. For example, if it occurs to me that the child has worked out that if he plays up he might keep his parents from splitting up, then I would wait for a convenient moment and start off by saying something like 'can I be devil's advocate' or 'would you mind if I put the cat amongst the pigeons'. Similarly if I get strong emotions when with a family or individual (or counter-transference if you prefer that term), I will usually share it or even act it out. For example, sometimes with families who are nice to each other and afraid of the boat being rocked, I may find myself wanting to say something that's maybe difficult to hear, but then back away from it because I feel too guilty about upsetting a family who have been nice to me. As soon as I realize this I might say 'I've just realized something which I've got to tell you', this might lead to a conversation about whether others in the family feel like I just felt. Sometimes I feel hopeless and don't know what to do to help someone and I share that. Sometimes I feel angry. This, I find, is a difficult emotion to talk about so often I just end up being angry and try to explain why. I guess transparency is part of deconstructing hierarchy. The more we hold secret knowledge as professionals, the more power we have over clients and I think the more vulnerable clients feel in our company.

Case vignettes

The following are a few short case vignettes, hopefully illustrating some of the points from the approach described above. Of course real life is much too varied, complicated, rich and diverse for us to simply apply a set of rules or principles in a uniform manner. The vignettes are based on real cases, real people's lives but with many of the details changed and with extracts from other cases being mixed in to each vignette in order to preserve confidentiality. Consent to publish these accounts was obtained from the parents of the main child in each of the following vignettes. My sincere thanks goes to these families who have allowed me to share some of their stories here.

Case I

David is the third born in a family of five children. He has an older brother and sister and two younger sisters. From early on in his school life he was noted to have learning difficulties, poor concentration, frequent loss of temper and aggression towards his peers. He was excluded from school on several occasions from his first year at primary school onwards. His mother became concerned and sought help from the local child and family consultation services. David was referred for child psychotherapy and attended this for a year. The family's perception was that the psychotherapy did not appear to make any significant difference to David's problems, particularly those at school. David's mother, Mrs A, then read an article about ADHD and discovered there was a local parent-support group whom she contacted. They encouraged her to seek help from a private clinic. The family then paid a lot of money to take David to this clinic. At this clinic David was diagnosed as having ADHD and started on Ritalin®. At this point David was 6½ years old. Mrs A, in describing the journey back on the train from this clinic, recalls feeling terribly guilty as she felt that previously she had been unaware that David was suffering from ADHD and to her this now meant that David did not have any control over his behaviour. Previously she had been trying to discipline him by telling him off. She had been telling him off for behaviours that she now felt David had no direct control over. At this clinic it was also suggested that David's father, Mr A, suffered from ADHD. Mr and Mrs A felt that this helped shed new light on the marital problems they had been having. They stopped taking David for psychotherapy, feeling let down by the local service which had not, in their view, picked up on the fact that David was suffering from ADHD. For the next couple of years David was much more settled in school. However, in response to telephone advice from the private clinic, the prescription of Ritalin® had been increasing in dose, until, by the time he was 9 years old, David was receiving a higher dose than Ritalin® is licensed for. Furthermore, many of the old problematic behaviours were re-emerging. David was no longer making any progress academically and he was requiring a lot of one-to-one support in the classroom. His attendance at school was around 70 per cent, partly because of days when the school requested he was taken home again, and partly because of days when Mrs A had decided not to send him to school for fear that he was going to be excluded. David's general practitioner then expressed his concern to the family about the dose of Ritalin® that David was on, particularly as he was concerned that David was now failing to gain height and weight adequately. At this point the school suggested that they return to the child and family consultation services, where they ended up being seen in our 'ADHD and other difficult to manage behaviours' clinic.

At the first session which was attended by David and Mrs A, there was a very strong emphasis on ADHD as the explanatory model, with Mrs A stating that to her it meant that David had a chemical imbalance in his brain. She mentioned that her husband had ADHD and that she also suspected her older son may have ADHD but that he had not yet been diagnosed. During this session she also, jokingly, said that maybe I had ADHD after I used a mild slang swear word when explaining something! The strong emphasis on ADHD at that time, I felt, was partly related to Mrs A's anxiety about returning to a service which she probably thought was skeptical about the diagnosis. She needed to test the waters and find out whether this new clinic was more in line with the, by now very strong, family belief that ADHD was the explanation for David's difficulties. I felt that we had to go with the flow and allow the family to engage. This meant taking a fairly chatty, open approach, acknowledging how difficult it must have been to come back to this service and being interested and curious to understand Mrs A's story about her experiences with different professionals. Within that chat we also started introducing a few ideas to deliberately complicate matters a little. We said things like 'of course there is a lot of disagreement amongst professionals about ADHD' as cues to get involved in early discussions about the meaning of the diagnosis.

We arranged a school visit, which showed us that the school too had been relying heavily on the idea of ADHD as an explanation, and that whenever David seemed to be having a bad day the first question was 'has he taken his medication'. The ADHD explanation had also allowed the school to become more sympathetic to David and his family's difficulties with him. This had meant that David was in the unusual position of being a child with quite low attendance but without an Education Welfare Officer being involved.

David himself was very defensive of, particularly, his mother in the early sessions. He found it hard to express his own ideas about what ADHD meant to him and what he felt about taking tablets, usually looking for help from Mrs A in answering questions.

Over the following months we tried to engage with the family by carrying out approximately once-monthly home visits. We also arranged a joint meeting with ourselves, Mrs A and the school head to try and find a better system to increase the amount of time David spent in school. The school also arranged for David to start attending an after-school club on certain days of the week. David began to increase the amount of time he was spending at school and, rather than sending him home on difficult days, the school, working together with the family, found a better alternative. This included allowing David a kind of positive time out where he was allowed to alert teachers, or teachers to alert him, that he was needing time out and he would go and spend some quiet time sitting in the head teacher's room.

Over the following year of sessions and intermittent crises the following, I think significant, part chance, part deliberate, things happened.

A number of alternative explanatory models began to emerge, volunteered spontaneously by the family, but it would have been very easy to miss or ignore their significance. Each time we heard such an alternative theory or story about David we would stop and try and follow it up, in an effort to bring this theory into the arena. At the same time we were slowly and repeatedly putting forward the idea that ADHD is a behavioural description not in itself an explanation. Alternative explanations included 'he has got a bad temper just like his father'. Engaging with Mr A was very important at this point and the home visits made this a lot easier. It led to some long discussions about temper and how it had affected Mr A's life, particularly as, according to him, he was thought to be a bright child who had under achieved. Mr A was so scared of his potential to lose his temper, having had a previous prison sentence when he was younger, that he had virtually locked himself in the house for fear that if he was outside he would be more likely to lose his temper, end up hurting somebody and getting another prison sentence. However, these stories also had important positive aspects which were very useful. Mr A had a lot of personal understanding about the problem of male tempers and its relationship to violence. He had a way of walking away from situations when he felt his temper was rising and would go and lock himself in one of the rooms in their house until he calmed down. This model, interestingly, had been picked up by David and without realizing it, at the time had been, I presume, part of the reason why David had suggested that when he was feeling angry he should go up to a teacher to ask for time out. Mr A was a family man and had struggled successfully to make sure his problem with tempers never resulted in any violence against any member of his family. He was clearly loved and respected by his children all of whom spoke up in defence of their parents. Mr A felt that these terrible tempers were part of the ADHD that affected him and that David had inherited. Consequently, after it was suggested at the private clinic that he also had ADHD, Mr A had eventually plucked up the courage to see a psychiatrist who put Mr A on anti-depressant medication. Mr A felt that the anti-depressant made him feel better, however, he still didn't feel able to mix socially or go for things like job interviews. The conversations about temper were also helpful as they led into more discussion of the overall family situation where, frequently, despite Mr A being available at home, it was Mrs A who took charge of issues such as discipline for all the children. This acted as a protection against Mr A losing his temper should the situation get heated, a position which often left Mrs A burdened with child care and sometimes guilty about feeling resentful at having to carry this burden for all the family. It also led to some discussions about the marital problems they had previously had and we were able to then talk about how important the ADHD diagnosis had been in saving their marriage and keeping the family together. Having these conversations and being able to share something about our own experiences of gender differences, with comments such as 'I sometimes feel like I could really lose it and get violent, whereas when my wife really loses it she ends up crying', helped humanize our relationship and I grew to like and respect this family a great deal.

Another alternative explanation occurred when a friend of theirs who was also in the house during one of our home visits, joined in the conversation and suggested that they made far more allowances for David than the other children. She felt that David was used to 'getting away with a lot more'. This led into a conversation about what happened after the diagnosis was given and how, at that time and since, they felt that David had no control over his behaviour, so that consequently they began making a lot more allowances for him. Mr and Mrs A were able to share their confusion about what the right thing to do is and how to judge what he does have control over and what he doesn't have control over. It was possible to introduce the idea that maybe David has some control over a lot more than they believe he has. This was partly confirmed in a later session when David, in relation to some question, offered another alternative explanation. He said that he liked being 'hyper' because when he was hyperactive he was the class clown and this was a time when other children laughed at him. For a child who had difficulty making friends this was an important way of getting some peer-group attention. Consequently, David admitted that sometimes when the nurse gave him the tablets at school he put them under his tongue and then threw them away. This was a bit of a shock, particularly for Mrs A, as she had to begin to revise her opinion concerning the degree of control David had over his behaviour.

Another useful alternative explanation was that David was born with learning difficulties and this has led him to feel frustrated when he feels he cannot achieve what other children are achieving. Thus, in this model his tempers are a sign of frustration and low self-confidence. This was an important explanation to follow up as it led to the whole issue of the tremendous amount of love and sympathy they have as a family towards David. Mrs A was open about how protective towards him she felt. Consequently, she was trying to protect him from trauma at school by keeping him away on days when she thought he would get in trouble. Unlike even his younger siblings, David was not allowed to go anywhere unescorted and therefore was unable to do things such as ride a bicycle even though his next younger sibling could. This gave an opportunity to collaborate with the family in drawing up a plan to increase David's independence step by step. This started with simple tasks such as escorting him to within 50 yards of the shop and then allowing him to go into the shop to buy something like a bottle of milk, or riding a bike on his own for 5 minutes just outside the house.

Another alternative explanation provided by the family was that David was the closest to his father. When we followed this up in a conversation there was an idea around that David was the one picking up his father's unhappiness, in other words sometimes David was an unhappy child and a sensitive child, picking up on the emotions going on around him. This also led to conversations about role models, copying and whether David himself wanted to be like his father.

With regard to medication, we managed to introduce successfully drug holidays, that is days and eventually the whole weekend off medication. Predictably, David was much more difficult to handle on those days; however, it felt important that the family also learned how to cope with him when he was off medication as well as when he was on it. Additionally, on the days off medication he ate much better and began gaining weight satisfactorily.

After a year, although we had not been able to bring down the dose of medication and the family still clearly believed in ADHD as an explanation; however, their beliefs were less rigid, complexity was more apparent in their thinking and they were taking their own ideas a little more seriously. David's school attendance was close to 90 per cent. He was more manageable at home and the overall family situation appeared to be improving. Mr A had started going for job interviews and mixing socially a little more. No miracles but a gradual engagement and the opening up of alternative avenues seemed to have resulted in a significant improvement. David and his family continue to be seen, after all a year later is still early days.

Case 2

Wesley was 8 years old when I first met him. He had been referred to our department several times previously and on each occasion the parents (Mr and Mrs G) had attended one or two appointments and then stopped coming. The G's are a working-class, east end of London family who express themselves openly and might seem intimidating if you're not used to having a little bit of contact with this sort of culture. They came complaining about how useless professionals are and demanding that something had to be done. They wanted to know if Wesley had this 'ADH thing' that somebody had mentioned to them (later I found out that it was Mr G's sister who had mentioned it as she had a son who had recently been diagnosed with ADHD). I felt my task in the first session was just to calm things down and I was able to pick up on a couple of things that seemed helpful in starting some sort of an engagement. First of all I picked up on Mrs G's idea that Wesley is like a disabled child and I felt that this was a useful idea to follow up. I agreed with her that, from what she had said, Wesley, although he looks perfectly normal, does appear to be somewhat disabled as he is unable to understand instructions and cannot concentrate for long periods, and in many ways he behaves like a much younger child. I also hoped that this would lessen some of the strong negative feelings Mr and Mrs G were expressing about Wesley. Second, I noticed that Mr G in particular liked to chat, so I happily engaged in chit-chat about all sorts of other things.

Next, I arranged a school visit where I got feedback that Wesley is quite a bright child, who seems to respond differently to different teachers. He seemed to know when he might get away with being more disruptive and when he wouldn't. He behaved quite well in his class with his class teacher who always maintained firm boundaries, but if there was a supply teacher who didn't know him, he could be terrible. He was noted to have problems concentrating, particularly during parts of the lesson when children were left to get on with a piece of work, where he seemed to lack focus, was easily distracted and often distracted others.

Next I carried out a home visit. Here I felt I was beginning to engage with the family, who were very happy for me to visit them so that they could show me all the damage Wesley had done at home. I followed up the idea of disability and fleshed this out by getting more descriptions of in what way they felt he was disabled and how this might affect him. I also began trying to look for the good news and to enquire about those times, however short, where Wesley was good. I also carried on chatting to Mr G about anything and everything. At the end of the initial assessment I described the different ADHD traits and the ones that Wesley had and did not have, and I suggested that according to the British system he would not be diagnosed as having ADHD but according to the American system he probably would. I also stated that his problems at home, diagnostically, were more of a conduct-disorder-type problem. The family seemed to take this, at this stage as meaning that Wesley did have ADHD and from thereafter referred to him as having ADHD. For most of the time I did not dispute this as it seemed to be helping them engage with a service that they had previously seen as useless. Initially, medication was not an issue for them as there were plenty of other things I was trying to help them with including meetings at school, moving house, getting child disability benefit and help with how to discipline Wesley. After a year of this sort of input there was no significant change in Wesley's behaviour and so at the request of the parents I discussed medication with them. We decided to start Wesley on Ritalin®. From the start Mr and Mrs G decided to follow my advice of having weekends without medication, and later also decided to take Wesley off medication during school holidays. Both school and home reported an immediate improvement, which proved a useful opportunity for everyone to see another side to Wesley. However after a year or so on Ritalin® the school requested a meeting which was attended by myself and Mrs G. They reported that Wesley seemed to be having problems with memory and many problem-solving exercises, where he often just sat staring at his book for long periods. This was particularly occurring during the first lessons in the morning and after lunch. The pattern seemed consistent with possible side effects from Ritalin® and Mr and Mrs G decided to take Wesley off it. The school reported an improvement in Wesley's memory and work thereafter with no noticeable deterioration in his behaviour. Mr and Mrs G didn't notice any deterioration in Wesley's behaviour either, on the contrary, they said that there seems to be the odd occasion now where he does appear to listen to them!

During these 2½ years, alternative explanations were also gradually building up. One of these was that Wesley is a child with lots of energy and that if he got more exercise he would not be so bad at home and would sleep better. However, the family were never able to organize it for him to be able to get regular exercise, and in some ways it was a vicious circle in that they wouldn't take him places for fear of how much he would play up in public.

At another session Mrs G briefly mentioned that Wesley 'had them wrapped around his little finger'. Having previously thought that they were quite strict, this was the first time I realized how often they gave in to Wesley. Both Mr and Mrs G were perfectly aware that this had negative consequences and were able to be open about how difficult it was for them not to give in to the 'anything for a peaceful life' temptation. I tried to support them in becoming more firm and consistent. I wrote a letter after that session urging them to stick with it when he got worse after they started not giving in.

Another useful explanation, which came from school and which I took up with the family was that Wesley is a bright child who uses his intelligence to work out how much he can get away with and with whom, and he is therefore different with different people as a result. This idea proved very useful in building stronger ties between the school and Mr and Mrs G (who agreed with this) and helped everyone think about how to get effective communication and consistency going between not only school and home, but also different teachers and different family members.

At another visit Mrs G told me that she did not get on with her father and explained that her father was very heavy handed with physical punishments. She had grown to fear him and hate him and still hated him to this day, even though he was now deceased. She was afraid that her children would grow up hating her in the same way that she grew up hating her father. Naturally, this led to a conversation about her feelings of guilt at any form of discipline and her worry that this may lead to her children disliking her.

After 2 years of working with Wesley and his family and just after Wesley was taken off Ritalin®, Mrs G expressed her honest doubts about the significance and meaning of the ADHD diagnosis. She said that she didn't understand 'where all this ADHD is coming from', it was not around when she was growing up but nowadays she keeps hearing of children who have got it. This led to a conversation about how different it is to be a parent nowadays compared to when she was growing up. She recalled how she and her siblings were able to go out and her parents were not concerned about where they went, providing they were back on time (which she frequently was not!). Nowadays she felt there was a constant fear about things such as drugs, bullying and even kidnapping. She felt sorry for her children, and Wesley in particular, whom she felt was an outdoor child. She felt parents these days cannot give their children the same degree of freedom as she and her siblings had in their childhood.

After 2½ years of working with them, Wesley and his family were, I believe, well engaged and the diagnosis of ADHD was hardly being talked about any more. They had been through various crises with home and school. They had lived through all of them and Wesley was no longer on medication. He had received a statement of special educational needs at school and was now making good progress, and although life continued to be a struggle for him and his family, there appeared to be good working relationships between the family and the agencies involved. They were coping with Wesley at home and were able to institute clearer boundaries. Tension at home had reduced and for the first time since I met them they were able to speak of good days occurring over a significant length of time.

Case 3

Jason attended for the first time together with his mother, Mrs B, when he was 7 years old. Mrs B is a single mother and Jason is the youngest of three children. He had learning difficulties, particularly in reading and writing but not so in activities like drawing and counting. He was very hyperactive when observed at school, in the clinic and at home, and had very poor concentration. Mrs B came across as a strong, determined, loving mother who wanted to get the best for Jason.

Initially, Mrs B was just curious to find out about ADHD. After the assessment was completed I was able to feed back that Jason clearly fulfilled the criteria for a diagnosis of ADHD. Medication was discussed and Mrs B made a definite decision not to put Jason on medication. Mrs B felt determined to find an alternative way to help Jason.

One of the first alternative stories to emerge was of Mrs B's own history of what she called dyslexia. She explained what happened to her at school, how she felt her reading and writing difficulties were never picked up and how she felt her poor reading and writing skills had knocked her confidence ever since. She felt Jason was like her in that respect and felt that he suffered from low self-confidence as a result. We worked with Jason's school and eventually Jason received a statement of special educational needs. I worked with Jason and Mrs B on his self-confidence discovering what he felt he couldn't do (and would then ruin) and what things he felt he could and was good at doing. Jason turned out to be a very lively, inventive, imaginative boy who was good at making things from all sorts of bits and pieces (toilet rolls, empty yogurt pots, cards, etc.). Mrs B started collecting stuff for Jason's creations and encouraged him a great deal with this. She also bought some educational toys (e.g. fridge-magnet letters, toy spelling computers) and made it a part of her daily routine to spend time with Jason working with these educational toys.

As her trust in me grew, Mrs B spoke more about her own difficult experiences and her realistic worries about how this may have affected Jason. She spoke about her postnatal depression and her worry that she had neglected Jason during this time. She spoke about Jason's father and how, prior to her running away from him to a women's refuge, Jason had witnessed a terrifying ordeal where his father had hit Mrs B and kept her prisoner for several hours before leaving their house. I just made a point of listening to her concerns and worries and not necessarily reassure her as to the possible effects these things had on Jason, as I felt she was trying to convey a deep sense of real understanding as to the effects such difficult experiences have on people and their relationships. Soon after that Mrs B started telling me that she was trying to be more patient with Jason and had been listening to him and his explanations and trying herself to explain more things to him. She also reported that she had become much firmer with him and seemed to be getting somewhere with this, at the same time as feeling that she was communicating much more with Jason and understanding him much better.

By 2 years down the line, Jason was no angel but was doing much better at school and home. School reported that he still had difficulty concentrating and settling to tasks, but that he was no longer aggressive, was making friends and they no longer classed him as a child with behavioural problems, his statement of educational needs being based on his learning difficulties. Mrs B felt her relationship with Jason had improved enormously over the past 2 years. She was no longer concerned or preoccupied with Jason's diagnosis of ADHD and felt much more reassured that his future was not going to be a mirror of hers. She felt that his strengths lay in his hands and his practical abilities and that all she wanted to be sure about was that when it comes to his adult life that he would be able to read and write and to respect others.

Chapter 8

Changing my practice: incoporating cultural diversity and a post-modern perspective

So I came to realize that what I had been taught and trained in was a faith, a belief system, a system of values, a way of judging people, pathologizing people, a way of developing and maintaining certain social behaviours and practices, a way of defining conformity and deviance, a way of liberating you if you believed and could opt into these values, a way of terrorizing you if you couldn't, a way of upholding the economic system, a way of jollying you up by changing your thinking or chemically manipulating your brain so that you can return to the misery that drove you over the edge, a way of colluding with the elite, the snob, the colonizer, a way of joining a fraternity, of belonging, a way of changing, a way of staying the same, a way of life.

But what of this religion? Is it religion? Is it science? Or something in between? Does it matter? Scientists tend to explain unsolved scientific mysteries with their own particular interest. The whole science of psychiatry is based upon this explanation of scientifically unsolved mysteries according to the faith or belief system of the describer. To me it is a rather peculiar and soulless system for explanation. After all, many of our working definitions for the so-called mental illnesses we are apparently identifying, involve such deep mysteries as understanding how people define themselves. When we make a diagnosis of schizophrenia or manic depression, or even depression, we are, in effect, telling that person that everything they believe they are, and indeed their whole world view, is wrong and who they think they are, what they think their life is, is of no value, no importance, but is all generated by chemical reactions in their head. Not that I am saying that this view is always unhelpful, nor am I saying that this view has not been of comfort to many people at times of deep distress or retrospectively after this distress has passed, nor am I saying that psychiatrists always cynically wield such a view in a soulless, inhumane manner. For the psychiatrist who truly believes in this, his or her treatment will be a part of their compassionate attempt to help a fellow human being in accordance with what their faith has taught them. However, I still believe it is a rather soulless faith with a thin spirituality and, in its fundamentalist form (as with many other fundamentalist religions), likely to operate an authoritarian form of social control that marginalizes too many experiences.

During my training I found myself becoming more and more critical of the Arabic culture I grew up in. I do not now wish to see my childhood and adolescence through any rose-tinted spectacles as I continue to have many criticisms of many aspects of the Arabic culture I grew up in. However, I believe it was a fundamental failing of my training to have sold me a value system which effectively belittles the one I grew up with. In my psychiatry and psychotherapy training I was told that the culture I grew up with was more primitive, less psychologically minded, more cruel and barbarous and that women and children, in particular, from my culture had a hard time of it. Then I began to remember, we left Iraq just before the Iraq/Iran war began. My best friend in secondary school came up to me and for the first time my background, to him, was a plus because Iraq had attacked Iran and the then big enemy of the west, the Ayatollah. Iraq was a great hero nation. Then I learned that the western powers had been playing the usual games, that Sadam Hussein had been assisted into power in Iraq and that the CIA were providing Iraq with regular intelligence. Then the tables turned and Iraq became the big enemy. In the early hours of one morning I was woken up by a telephone call from my brother who told me to turn the television on. I watched the strangest form of media entertainment with live pictures of Baghdad being bombed. I have seen my father's extended family sent scattering, trying to escape the troubles, those strong extended family ties stretched to the limits as families and individuals have ended up peppered in different countries all over the world. Relatives have died, or been killed as a direct or indirect result of all that has happened in that region. I have heard that an estimated quarter of a million Iraqi children have died as a result of sanctions. A country, which once had a basic, but none the less present, system of education and health care and very basic welfare, has fallen apart with widespread malnutrition, disease and severe poverty. Iraq had tried to pick up the pieces after 40 years of British rule, but the west could not keep their hands off for very long. Now I wonder who is more primitive, less psychologically minded, more barbarous and more cruel to women and children?

In the end I did not have to go very far from home to start challenging the assumptions of my training. Which culture is it that is complaining about, for good reason, men who leave their families and their children, and bullying, violence, drug abuse, promiscuity, alcohol consumption (to name but a few) amongst the young. Which culture is it that is complaining about a lack of collectiveness amongst families, poor networks of support and a loss of morals and values? In which culture is it that selfish aims, greed and commodities have become the main way in which the value of your life is judged? Is this the sign of an advanced, psychologically minded, civilized, compassionate culture?

So, what of the science of psychiatry? Can we really take a dispassionate analysis of this as if it were a politically neutral, socially value-free enterprise? In psychiatry, science is more an illusion of science based on faith than anything else. There is a continual bugbear that psychiatry has been unable to overcome, which is that none of the apparently scientifically based hypotheses that underpin the whole system, has been validated in any concrete, material way. It is easy to list report after report during the last century of apparently clear findings confirmed by some and then refuted by others. In that sense there is convincing statistical, scientific evidence that the apparently convincing and confirmed findings will not be so in a little while. If psychiatry was following the basic scientific standards for verifying a hypothesis, then first there should be a description of something tangible, something that stands up to the tests required by medicine, of showing a physical cause and of coming to an understanding about what this cause might be. It must also show that the symptoms occur amongst a group of people for reasons other than chance and that there is some kind of underlying, unifying process at work. By this benchmark psychiatry has thus far proven itself not to be a scientific discipline. Yet it is often ruled by a fundamentalist belief that it is. Because faith comes in we have some unsustainable beliefs in the power of science. We believe schizophrenia, depression, obsessive compulsive disorder, and so on must exist because science says it does and if science says it does then it must be so and because these are without a doubt scientific concepts they must, by implication, be beyond challenge. It must be a truth. It is beyond criticism because it is scientific, therefore to criticize these concepts would be unscientific. This is the circular argument that the fundamentalist position is effectively maintaining.

In this scientific bible there are certain commandments that must be followed and seen as the highest order in which quality knowledge can be derived.

Take, for example, the double-blind clinical trial. This is very often quoted as the gold standard by which treatment can be evaluated, and is the approach that is employed in the rest of medicine, particularly for trials in assessing the effectiveness of medication. The double-blind trial works something like this: let us assume a drug which I will call A is about to be tested on those with a diagnosis of a disorder that I shall call X. When the trial commences half of those with the diagnosis X will be given drug A and the other half will be given drug B, which the new drug A is being compared with. The medication will be manufactured as far as possible so that those with diagnosis X will not know whether they are on drug A or drug B, furthermore the clinician prescribing the medication will also not know whether their patient is receiving medication A or medication B. The procedure is called double blind because two people, the person with the diagnosis and the prescribing clinician, do not know (in other words are blind) whether the patient is receiving medication A or medication B.

The fundamentalist maintains that the double-blind clinical trial is the gold standard for evidence-based treatment. In some ways this makes sense. If we were dealing with known medical conditions, and consequently treatments that had some rational basis in material reality, then the double-blind clinical trial would make some sense, at least for the medical component of any disorder. However, the reality is that this type of trial, which is the gold standard for the rest of medicine, is miserably out of place in psychiatry. This is where the fundamentalist system of appraising evidence really comes unstuck and where the massive gap between research-based views of mental life and clinical reality becomes evident. The fundamentalist researcher following his/her faith in the pursuit of pure knowledge, works with select motivated groups in artificial settings ruled by unidimensional linear ideas. She/he produces findings which are either of little use to the everyday clinician who deals with unmotivated groups, people who drop out of treatment, multi-problem situations and, in this day and age, wide complex belief systems and for whom the psychological factors (which are seen as something that should be eliminated in a pure double-blind, randomized trial) are an important part of the 'bread and butter' of helping clients. Then of course there is the problem of how you interpret the findings. Given the lack of a material starting point, the significance of any finding is fitted around a belief system so that the interpretation of the relevance of the finding is always coloured by the interpretation frame-work into which it is fitted. So I have learned to cast a critical eye on the basic methodology of research in psychiatry. It has been imported wholesale from medicine but without a material starting point on which to base the research and interpret its findings. It is a mistake to believe that pure empiricism will unravel the subjective, this fundamentalist position is unsustainable. I have learned that belief systems are inescapable and that findings are interpreted according to belief systems as there is no other material reference point to use. In some ways it is not surprising to find that trying to establish some sort of truth and certainty about subjective life takes us straight back into subjective life again.

Once I had learned to question the values and beliefs of this psychiatric, mental-health culture and began to realize that the truth which its priests preach was as shaky and subjective as all the other historical claims to have found truth, I felt anger (anger at having the wool pulled over my eyes, anger at being cultured into this, anger at not seeing through it earlier, anger at being socialized into condemning and distancing myself from the values and beliefs which I grew up with, which are a part of my heritage, which are important to me and a part of that thin sense of belonging that somewhere I still possessed). I felt scared, I did not want to be an outsider, I did not know how far I could challenge the system and survive within it, I did now know how far I could be allowed to change. I did not want to become some crazy maverick, inventing ways of practicing *ad hoc*. I still wanted to be able to pay the mortgage.

And then, of course, you find yourself tracking back. Maybe I was wrong, maybe I was being unfair, progress is being made all the time and maybe we all need to be more patient with the science of psychiatry, even though it has not delivered the goods yet it will only be a matter of time before it does so. Progress, now there's a word that comes up again and again in our culture. In fact, it is very central to the whole idea behind science as a faith. This knowledge that we are gaining about the world is progress, progress means that life is becoming better for all of us. It means we are moving in the right direction. I come back to the big picture. Progress for whom and in what way. Okay, we have become technically capable, we are better able to protect ourselves from nature, we live longer (the lucky ones in this world that is), the fortunate among us can protect ourselves against physical unpleasantness and increase physical pleasure in our lives. Is that progress? My suspicion is that on those scores more than half of the world would probably disagree, they have not seen any of it. For them progress has meant a refinement of the ways of being exploited, tortured and brutalized.

But what of that other source of suffering, the social suffering that Freud referred to (see Chapter 3)? Have we made progress there? I agreed with Freud that every culture struggles with this one. Each culture comes up with a set of beliefs, values and rules to try and reduce this suffering (psychiatry is part of our culture's way of dealing with it). But progress? Has this culture really got anywhere with social suffering, has psychiatry got anywhere with mental pain? I don't think so. In fact I want to be bold enough to ask if our culture, psychiatry and all, has lost something very valuable about human life with this tyranny of progress. Bound by the gods of consumerism there is a quest for knowledge as though it was a fundamental need in this religion of science. To satisfy the need for faith and for economic survival we must continue to produce knowledge. Knowledge is power they say. Is knowledge this culture's form of enlightenment? It seems in this culture that reaching enlightenment is about reaching the pinnacle of Maslow's pyramid where apparently self-realization occurs (Maslow, 1987).

This is where I think the faith of science misses out. It is about a quest for knowledge, which is devoid of spirituality, devoid of a sense of connection to bigger realities, to the earth, to the natural world, to history, to context, to each other. In many other cultures wisdom is not just about knowledge, it's not about collecting data (there's a difference between knowledge and knowing). Enlightenment is not about a selfish, materialistic self-realization. This is where I believe our culture misses out. The gods we worship, such as money and material goods, are frivolous and empty yet we worship them even though we think we don't. Has meaning in our lives come to revolve around shallow, material things? Still that is the way things are. I have often wondered whether there may be such a thing as a science of faith, in the sense that having faith, believing in something is a fundamental human necessity without which our lives become meaningless and purposeless. If this is the case then it seems to me likely that the practice of psychiatry and, indeed, any practice geared towards mental-health problems, will always be steeped with ideas and beliefs derived from what I am calling a faith, just as this book is in some ways an expression of my faith, my beliefs. Perhaps in this particular time when faith and meaning has become rather thin, it's no surprise to see this, in some general way, reflected in a lingering, widespread unhappiness and a parallel rise in the number of professionals dealing with mental-health difficulties. Psychiatrists and a whole range of therapists and counsellors are maybe trying to give this individualistic society some sense of cohesion to hold the society together and keep alive networks which have meaning and substance.

So, with the help of respected colleagues I began to move beyond the assumptions that had dominated the way I had worked.

The following then represents a very brief look at a few of the issues and approaches I have thought about and begun using since starting to challenge the assumptions of my training and changing my practice. The list is not meant to reflect a systematic way of categorizing the mental-health problems that we deal with (as, for example, psychiatry attempts to do). The list is born out of personal reflections that come out of clinical experience and it reflects an attempt to move out of a way of defining mental-health problems that is arrived at through the illusion of objectivity. Instead I have moved into the territory of subjectivity that, I believe, dominates this field of human experience. The challenging of dominant assumptions does not mean falling into an anarchic, free-for-all, crazy therapy. It is a shame that I have to mention this at this point, as so frequently I have encountered colleagues who react to something that is different, that is outside their understanding of psychiatric culture, as being deviant and inevitably crazy. Recently an adult psychiatric colleague of mine commented to me after a presentation I did on alternative approaches: 'so if you are lying on the roadside after an accident with a broken leg you would not be asking for an aromatherapist?' Implicit in this sort of comment is the idea that you lose touch with reality when you attempt to move away from the dominant assumptions. Neither is this approach attempting to discard the idea that there are universals, in other words principles, behind our human functioning that are applicable to all. However, the more you challenge the dominant assumptions within mental health the harder it becomes to know where these universals lie and what their boundaries are (my experience has led me to believe that many, if not most, of the universals that mental-health professionals believe in are, in fact, better understood as cultural impositions).

What it has meant is recognizing the culturally tinted glasses that we all wear as professionals, and that has a massive influence on the way we practice. It has meant trying to take off these glasses and discovering other ways of understanding mental-health problems and their solutions, and rehabilitating these back into the melting pot of our theories and our practice. It has meant decreasing the relative importance of my professionally derived systems of explanation and increasing the importance of the client-derived systems of explanation (what some call local knowledge), the ordinary, the human, the intuitive. What I believe has happened is largely a change in my attitude towards the knowledge systems I am familiar with. It has resulted in challenging the hierarchy and recognizing the man-made (as opposed to the naturally occurring) nature of our frameworks. It has meant opening my mind to using other systems of knowledge. As my practice has changed I have not attempted to generate new knowledge nor have I discarded the current knowledge available. Thus the following represents a brief description of how my change in attitude has affected the way I work around a number of issues. I have deliberately avoided cluttering up the text with references. Changes are subtle, complex, human processes with all sorts of influences such as colleagues, family and clients, who probably have had a bigger influence on this process than any text(s) I have read.

Incorporating post-modern therapies

I have found many of the therapy ideas that have come out of the post-modern approaches to human problems refreshingly simple yet insightfully complex in a way that leaves plenty of scope for that important subjective creativity. It has allowed me to be an ordinary person in my professional life and freed me from the baggage and weight of unjustifiable assumptions that accompany my professional title.

Narrative approaches

My understanding of the 'narrative therapy' approach, is that it emphasizes the importance of the stories we are surrounded by (about ourselves and our world), in their influence on how we attribute meaning to the events of our lives (including of course, the problems we encounter). Our identities develop in this melting pot of stories about our world and about us, as told by the many different influential voices in our lives. Therapy revolves around the idea of joining the client/family in developing a new 'script' (or more usually re-invigorating an old, potentially helpful, story), usually one that enlarges on the strengths and competencies of the client/family and that can change some of the meaning being attributed to a problem in a way that frees up the client/family's own resources to solve that problem. When I see clients and their families, they usually have come to tell me about a problem and so I get a 'problem-saturated' account of the young person I have been asked to see. The challenge is to look for, and bring out, the functional, positive aspects about the client as a way of developing a more positive set of identities for him/herself, as well as developing the functional and positive aspects of the family's problem-solving abilities. In some ways this reminds me of Unani (or Tibb) medicine's emphasis on strengthening an ill person's natural healing capacity.

I saw a 7-year-old boy called Steven Saunders. His general practitioner, mainly because of the school's concerns, had referred him. In a letter from Steven's head teacher, she said that in her 20 years of teaching she had never come across a child as unruly and bizarrely behaved as Steven. On entering the consulting room a very moody Steven decided he wouldn't speak to me. His upset parents told me he didn't want to come as he thought he was going to be in even more trouble. I commended them on their sensitive understanding of the possible reason behind Steven's moodiness, which allowed us a conversation of how they felt Steven was unhappy at school as he was always blamed for any trouble and in their opinion had given up trying. Steven sat drawing Pokemon (cartoon characters) pictures. After a while I went and crouched next to him telling him that I'd been watching him and was amazed at how carefully he had drawn his picture and how good it was. We spoke about Pokemon for a bit and then he wrote his name at the top of his picture in beautiful handwriting and I commented on how beautifully he wrote. His parents were amazed and told me his school thought he couldn't write his name. I joined in with the parent's version of events and agreed that maybe Steven had simply lost the motivation to try because of unhappiness at school. I then made an audiotape and sent this to Steven. The tape had a story on it that I made up about a character I called 'Super Strong Steven Saunders' who hated school and every time he tried to change no one noticed. In the story he is visited by a fairy godfather who keeps reminding him to try and warns him that it will take time before others notice. This fairy godfather knows he can do it because he's been watching him and knows he isn't called Super Strong Steven Saunders for nothing. I attended a school review meeting for Steven several months later. He had settled in class, was no longer disruptive, had caught up academically and was regularly earning merits for good behaviour.

I saw a 15-year-old boy called Daniel who had previously been diagnosed with autism. He was in trouble at school for fighting back when other boys teased him. He had no friends and had recently been 'rubbing' himself against girls at school. At the first meeting with the family which was understandably dominated by a 'because of his autism' set of explanations, I had an opportunity to stop the conversation when his mother mentioned that when Daniel was much smaller he had seemed to know when she was upset. I showed a lot of interest in this and by highlighting and punctuating our conversation here, I felt I had an opportunity to re-open a long-buried (by the diagnosis) line of thinking that took us out of the autism frame. I found out about how upset Daniel was about the breakup of his parents' relationship, although he often hid this. I found out that in the aftermath of the breakup, Daniel would often come up to his mum and ask if she was all right. When she was feeling down sometimes he would come up and cuddle her spontaneously. I kept saying things like 'that's really interesting', 'what a sensitive boy' and 'that doesn't fit in with autism'. I watched Daniel's body language move from disinterested disengagement to furtive glances at his mother and downward embarrassed glances. He was listening. His mum also said that sometimes she'd wondered whether it is autism or something else. I suggested that it was possible that Daniel is a sensitive child who had built a protective bubble around him to shield him from pain that he feels deeply sometimes. I also suggested that this bubble could make him look like he's autistic. This seemed to make sense to Daniel's mum who started mentioning other bits of behaviour here and there that didn't fit in, for her, with autism. He loves animals ('really? how sensitive'). He plays cricket on Saturdays and is well respected by the other players ('wow, so when he doesn't have to worry too much about rejection, he's perfectly capable of mixing with other children' etc.). Over the following sessions the more we spoke about Daniel's competence and the well-functioning side of his life, the more animated he became. Six months later, Daniel was experiencing no behavioural problems in school, had made friends (including a friend of the opposite sex), was planning his career and was no longer 'moody' at home. He had become increasingly able to chat in our sessions. At his request I wrote to his general practitioner and school saying that Daniel does not have a diagnosis of autism.

I saw a 13-year-old boy called Gary. He had developed severe, crippling obsessions and compulsions that had stopped him from attending school. He was admitted to an adolescent unit where his obsessions and compulsions reduced and almost disappeared, only for them to re-appear on discharge home, which was the point when I first met him and his parents. Gary and his parents were feeling very defeated. I decided to give the obsessions and compulsions a persona. I called it a bully and started a conversation about how he had shown how normal he was when he went to the unit, but returned home to find this bully still there. I asked them how the bully affects their lives, what it stops each of them from doing, what would they be doing if the bully wasn't there, how have they fought the bully in the past, what has worked even if just for a minute and so on. I picked up on small successes and small things that were different since being discharged from the adolescent unit. I suggested that they had already started fighting back against the bully. I suggested they pick one situation in which to battle against the bully. They picked the night-time rituals and checks, kept a diary and went into battle. That was about 8 months ago. Gary has been back in school full time for about 5 months. He now does very occasional minor checks that are no different to the ones most of us do.

Solution-focused approaches

The solution-focused approach offers a more structured method of trying to achieve similar goals to the narrative approach, that of developing the functional healthy aspects of the clients and their families (as opposed to getting rid of the patho-logical, ill, dysfunctional aspects). The basic idea, as I understand it, is that after joining with the client/family through chat and listening to their story (usually a problem-saturated story), you ask the client/family what it is that they would like to see change, to see different in their lives. This can be helped along by questions like the miracle question 'Imagine you woke up tomorrow and for some reason, you don't know how or why, but a miracle had happened and everything you want to change in your life, had changed. What would tomorrow be like? What would be different about it? What's the first thing you would notice that's different?', or the crystal ball question 'If I had a crystal ball and could look into the future and see you in 6 months time after all your wishes had come true, what would I see?', or for younger children three wishes 'If I could grant you three wishes to change anything you want, what would your three wishes be?' A list of desired changes or goals to work towards can then be developed. The current situation can then be 'rated', by asking the client/family to give a score out of ten for how things are at the moment, where zero is none of the things in the list of goals ever happens and ten is they happen all the time. If they don't score themselves at zero then you can start a conversation about the exceptions, in other words the instances where, even if briefly, the client/family are already achieving something from their list of goals. If zero or under (it does happen!) is scored, you can go through the list again carefully looking for exceptions (they nearly always exist) or start a conversation about coping mechanisms (e.g. 'Zero, god that's dreadful, how do you cope? How did you manage to get yourself here today? Even though it's zero you still dressed well for today, amazing', etc.). At the end of the session you can set a small task, perhaps one thing from the list that the client/family have decided to work on first. You can ask a question like 'Can you think of one thing you could do that's different to what you do at the moment that might make a small difference and improve your score just a little bit for this goal?' By focusing on anything that has changed, even just a tiny bit or for a short while, in subsequent sessions, you can start building a more positive, functional view of the problem and the client/family's own abilities to solve it. I often use metaphors like 'If you try to get to the top of a flight of stairs by jumping, you'll probably keep falling back to the bottom, best to try a step at a time'. I also try and slow down expectations for change by using the 'old habits die hard' metaphor. To try and anticipate setbacks I use metaphors like 'better the devil you know than the devil you don't' to suggest that changing your emotional life can be quite scary.

I saw a 16-year-old girl called Reehana. She came with her mother and they told me that Reehana had been losing weight and refusing to eat meals with them for the past 6 or so months and that in the past 2 weeks she had got visibly worse. Her weight-for-height ratio when I first saw her was around 70 per cent of the normal. I did the miracle question with Reehana and her list included things like feeling happier and having more confidence. I asked her how would she and other people know if she was happier or more confident, what would she be doing. Her list became more specific to include things like talking with and going out with her friends, watching her brother at his football games and singing along to music at home. I asked her if these things had been happening more or less commonly since this weight-loss thing got control of her. She said less commonly. This gave me the opportunity to suggest to her that 'anorexia' saw that she was vulnerable and had been selling her false promises of happiness and self-confidence, but in reality had been doing a good job of trying to control her in such a way that her chances of happiness and self-confidence were getting further and further away. She seemed to see what I was saying and from then on it was relatively straightforward to work with her, session by session, setting new goals for her. She began eating, socializing, developing her interests and made a complete physical and mental recovery.

Incorporating culture

This is a big subject that goes well beyond looking at, respecting and working with the beliefs and practices of other cultures. It means being able to look at differences within our own culture (e.g. class, location and politics). In particular it means being able to cast a critical eye over our professional culture and question many of its assumptions. I have used various sub-headings to try and give some order to my thoughts.

Professional identity

As a medical student I was once told to smarten up my appearance by a senior doctor (the top button on my shirt was undone) who explained to me that as a doctor I was joining an exclusive club and had to learn to look the part. I also remember being told off as a junior doctor working in a child-psychiatric department, for wearing suede shoes. The consultant explained to me that the paediatricians wouldn't respect another doctor who does not look the part. Throughout my psychiatric training there has been a slow 'drip drip' of messages from senior colleagues about the importance of cutting off your feelings, keeping a calm and controlled exterior and not getting emotionally involved in clients' problems. There are cultural expectations about being a doctor and professional etiquette. It is interesting to contrast this with how little attention has been given to the importance of such notions as compassion, humanity and listening to the voice of users. The message that built up was that my professional identity should be a boundaried, protected and separated identity, allied to my role as a technician. Although never comfortable in this role, this idea of the professional identity of the mental doctor had a strong influence on the way I practiced in my earlier years. As I reached my turning points and met a number of practitioners whose notion of professional identity was radically different, I found myself slowly taking off my white coat and my professional self became less and less separated from my personal self.

Nowadays, I am more interested in the everyday issues, in the importance of the ordinary, in small talk and chat, in warmth and friendliness, in being transparent (in other words theorizing with the clients rather than developing private theories to share with a circle of colleagues that excludes the client). I like humour, light-heartedness, expressing my own emotions, saying how something makes me feel and showing my feelings (e.g. getting into a passionate argument with a client). I try to be honest which sometimes means painful straight talking. I like to share information from my own life, from my family's life and allow people to be nosey about me in the same that I am being nosey about them. I can be defensive sometimes, feel comfortable using intuition (as opposed to reason), allow awkward silences to happen and cover up for awkward silences. My work self is more similar to the self in the rest of my life. I have a mixture of pleasant and unpleasant experiences with my clients, a mixture of people who take to me or don't, who I take to or don't, a mixture of experiences that reflect the inherent simplicity and complexity of relationships. Perhaps one of the most important shifts, as I have changed my attitude to my work, is that of greater openness and transparency. All the theories and emotions and intuitions that I had previously kept private I now view as public property to be put into the melting pot of the session.

Perhaps the person you are in any mental-health treatment is more important than what you do. I remember a child-psychiatric consultant who I worked for who was particularly against the psychoanalytic model. In her criticism of psychoanalytic psychotherapy she told me about how, as a young trainee, she was considering going for personal therapy. She visited a number of therapists and discovered that the therapists with a good reputation seemed to be those who were the most pleasant to meet. She was putting this forward as a way of criticizing psychoanalytic psychotherapy, saying that the outcome was probably a function of the quality of the therapist as opposed to the quality of the therapeutic technique. My interpretation would be that this is so for all of the therapies and that it is further confirmation that in the subjective practice of problems in subjective life, the type of person a therapist is with their clients has a big influence on outcome.

The assessment/treatment split

Treatment starts the minute an assessment starts and as you are carrying out treatment you are constantly getting new information which is changing, or at least updating your assessment of the situation. Psychiatric training teaches you to put a boundary between an assessment and a treatment. Whilst this man-made boundary may be helpful in certain situations (e.g. requests for a professional opinion from another agency to whom you are handing your client back) this split does not reflect the way processes naturally develop in a relationship (including the professional/ client relationship). Of course the different theoretical orientations teach different ways of conducting an assessment. A family therapist may ask to meet with the family and focus on obtaining different views and observing the interactions between family members. A psychodynamic psychotherapist may focus on first impressions of the client's interactions with them for clues to the emotional make up and possible conflicts within the client. As a child psychiatrist you are also taught a certain ritualisatic method for conducting your assessments. This involves taking a history in a manner similar to the rest of medicine. You start by collecting information about the presenting problem and obtaining a developmental, social, medical and family history. Then there is some degree of check-listing, checking whether the client takes drugs or alcohol, has suicidal ideas, eating, sleeping and activity levels and so on. There may be a physical examination of the child. However, the biggest emphasis in the psychiatric assessment is on the, so-called, mental-state examination. This is the examination that the psychiatrist is meant to be conducting during the assessment interview to give them a symptom profile for the client. During the interview the psychiatrist is noting down things such as delusions, thought disorder (e.g. jumbled-up sentences, jumping topics with no apparent connection), hallucinations such as auditory hallucinations, the quality of the client's speech, activity level in the client, any tics or other abnormal movements, impulsivity, the quality of interaction with others in the room, and so on. According to our textbooks and the exams we take, in about an hour we should be able to complete a psychiatric assessment on any individual and arrive at a provisional diagnosis. In child psychiatry this ritual assessment inevitably also involves meeting the child's carers and is based primarily on the information provided by them.

The assessment ritual in child psychiatry keeps the psychiatrist reassured about their medical identity. Like many other models it squeezes the complex human processes that we deal with into a particular, rather narrow, rigid framework for understanding and dealing with it. By providing a diagnosis, the psychiatrist (and often the parents and referrer) feel they have something concrete and that a definite understanding of a problem has been developed. The medical label can have a very powerful, often hypnotic, effect on everyone, channelling the meaning given to the situation into a unidimensional, easy-to-understand frame. Although this frame may prove helpful (at least for a while), the reality is that very little can have been understood through applying medical labels with no accompanying medical facts to back them up.

I have moved away from this, limiting, inhibiting and essentially dishonest psychiatric model, although of course I have the advantage that all this and other models are sitting in the back of my mind and, to some degree, are accessible to me during a session. However, I have found that the simple things like common human courtesy, warm careful listening, up-front honesty, and a transparency regarding my thinking (sharing ideas as they arrive in my head) are enough to engage most families in a way that feels comfortable, meaningful, yet fairly ordinary and day-to-day. Where I believe that diagnosis might have an unhelpful, killing effect on the capacity to include other potentially useful avenues for exploration, I try and move a first meeting away from this. Psychiatric diagnosis can very easily be 'deconstructed', for example by stating 'A psychiatric diagnosis really just describes behaviour, it's not like other medical diagnoses like, say, pneumonia, where I can listen with a stethoscope or take an x-ray. There are no tests I can do to help us know what's wrong with him/her and so any diagnosis he gets doesn't tell us why he/she has something physical wrong with him/her, nor does it tell us what to do about the problem, it's just a convenient way of describing some of his/her behaviour'. I am very comfortable with engaging in debate, discussing controversies and answering questions as best as I can. I find this process of deconstructing particularly important with the many clients I see who have seen different doctors and been given different diagnoses for their child. In the early sessions I do not see it as my task to carry out a mental-state examination and arrive at a diagnosis (unless there is a particular reason to do so), but rather to find out what the expectations of the clients are, what they hope to get out of coming to see me and to look for early opportunities to try an intervention.

The first meeting is often a golden opportunity for an intervention that can sometimes have very powerful effects.

I met with a single mother and her three children for the first time. She told me about how her oldest son was very challenging and how he and his brother were constantly having fights that sometimes resulted in injury and that she was too scared to stop. She told me about their horrendous history which included domestic violence, being married unknowingly to a paedophile, her own childhood of sexual abuse and so on. She looked very down and hopeless as if she felt destined for their lives to always go wrong. I kept repeating about what a remarkable women she was, how not only had she the strength and courage to survive the most difficult of circumstances, but she had also shown her love and determination to do what she believed was best for her children whenever any of these awful things happened. I suggested many less-able people would have collapsed under this stress by now. I wrote a letter after this appointment reiterating this. I saw them again 3 months later. The children were being well managed, the fighting at home had stopped, and their mum had given up a 20-year habit of smoking and had started working with a voluntary organization, something she had always wanted to do. They did not request a further appointment so I told them I would leave the case open for 6 months in case they wished to see me again. After 6 months they were contacted and were happy to be discharged.

I met with a 16-year-old girl who had become distressed, tearful, not sleeping, withdrawn, self-harming and preoccupied with death since a year previously when she had had an operation for a burst appendix. In the first session she told me that she believed she should have died, that somehow she had cheated fate by surviving. She had been misdiagnosed when she first presented to her doctor with stomach pain and later had to be rushed to hospital for an urgent operation after her appendix had burst. She was told she was lucky to be alive. She suffered from some complications after her operation and needed a prolonged stay in hospital. At the first meeting I engaged her in a long conversation about fate, sharing my opinion that fate had obviously meant her to survive. I asked her to start socializing with her friends again and to make a point of looking at her scar every morning and afternoon whilst telling herself 'I survived', until she was bored with doing that. Three months and two appointments later she was happy, mixing and socializing, sleeping well and said that her scar had now faded and she hardly ever thought about it.

Parenting

The job of parenting has become the intellectual property of professionals. Apparently passed-on wisdom is no longer good enough, it is the professionals who know best when it comes to the question of how to rear children. From Doctor Spock to your health visitor, professionals know best. I point this out, not to condemn professional knowledge as useless, but to challenge the assumption that professional opinions are necessarily the best. Furthermore, it must be appreciated that current professional thinking on child rearing is based not on scientific universals, but on a fundamentally modernist, western, cultural-value system that emphasizes individuality and freedom of expression for children. Values such as family loyalty, obedience to parents, responsibility towards younger siblings and the community are no longer central. In this atmosphere the message sent out to parents is that children should all be treated as individuals, encouraged to express themselves, have voices, develop self-control and be a little like small adults with the same rights. When my son was coming up to a year old my wife was heavily pregnant with our second child. I took my son for his developmental check with the health visitor. With no prompting the health visitor told me to expect my son to be jealous after his sibling was born and told me 'I should sit him down and talk to him about us having a new baby soon' (my son could only understand a few simple instructions)!

Boundaries between the parents and their child are also emphasized. This shows itself in many ways. For example, there exist the professional beliefs that children should not be encouraged to sleep in the same bed as their parents and that children should not be given any form of physical chastisement (as this is believed to violate a physical boundary around the child). On the nurturing side, the style that appears to be encouraged in western culture is one that involves the use of verbal expression (compared to physical ways of expressing yourself which are more common in many cultures centred around the family as the primary social unit). The importance of play and stimulation is also emphasized. Talking to your children, a lot of eye contact and overt verbal expressions of love, caring and praise, playing with your children, plenty of toys and so on, appears to be the order of the day.

If we look at those cultures where the family is the primary social unit there are a number of important differences in the emphasis placed within the cultural values for parenting. There is often an emphasis on a sense of responsibility and obligation for parents (both cultural and religious), furthermore, this sense of obligation and responsibility to the family is passed on to the children. In this sort of set up the needs and desires of the individual child take second place to the needs of the family unit. The sense of boundaries exist less so around the individual and more so around the family. In many family-orientated cultures you see a much greater blurring of boundaries between parent and child with dependence being allowed to fully express itself in young children. For example, it is more common to see children being encouraged to sleep with their parents, physical chastisement and more physical as opposed to verbal expressions of love and affection. At the same time it is arguable that the notion of responsibility and obligation leads to a different sort of boundary between parents and children with more emphasis on the role of parents to protect children from unhappiness and discomfort.

The more hands-off as opposed to hands-on approach valued by western professionals is reflected in the way many of our institutions operate. Salim was 13 years old when I first met him. He had come, with his family, from Pakistan a couple of years earlier. His school was complaining to his parents that he was not doing his homework and was falling far behind, despite being a capable lad. The school believed this was because he was unhappy. The parents explained that, in their opinion, Salim was doing this because he could. In Pakistan, there wasn't a problem with him doing his homework. Here however, he wasn't filling in his homework book and as far as they could see there was no punishment from the school for him not doing his work. They believed that if his teachers would fill in his homework book, they would be able to check that he's doing it. I arranged a meeting at the school. They told us that Salim's punishment was detention, but that he was not attending his detentions (i.e. that Salim had to take responsibility for making sure that his punishments were administered!). I asked the school if they could, as Salim's parents had suggested, arrange for his teachers to fill in his homework book at the end of each lesson. The school initially insisted that this was not possible, not only for practical reasons, but also because it ran counter to their philosophy that someone of Salim's age should be encouraged to take responsibility for his actions. They believed that the measure we were suggesting would encourage unhealthy dependency that was inappropriate at his age. After much arguing about this cultural ideal, the school eventually agreed to the request. Within a couple of weeks, Salim was completing all homework and achieved excellent exam results at the end of that academic year.

Farooq was 8 years old when a colleague and I first met him together with his Algerian father. Farooq sat on his chair, didn't play with the toys in the room and answered questions politely and respectfully. My white, western colleague was concerned by this behaviour, feeling that Farooq was not showing normal childhood curiosity or playfulness, and was being too deferential to his father. She was concerned that his father may be physically or emotionally abusing him, to the extent that Farooq was now terrified of his father. My opinion was that Farooq was a credit to his father and was probably being raised with a strong sense of a cultural-value system that emphasizes the importance of respecting your elders.

I have often wondered whether our professional preoccupation with play, stimulation and hands-off guidance, results in what might be considered over-stimulating environments. These days I often deliberately put away all the toys in the consulting room when first meeting a child who has been referred because the child is (in the opinion of the referrer) hyperactive, to see how they behave in a non-stimulating environment (as well as to create a non-distracting environment which I find is better for starting the process of engaging a child).

There are many other social and political realities that have a massive impact on the way we parent. Living in a capitalist market economy where religious values have become increasingly marginalized, means having to live with the fact that children are now regarded as potential consumers targeted by all sorts of advertising. This, no doubt, results in families having to live with children who demand material things. Protecting children from early sexual awareness has become a very difficult task with so many sexual images that are easily accessible, and with sex being talked about at younger and younger ages in schools and amongst peer groups (it is the same with gruesome, violent, horror images). Income and class-related issues also have an important impact. The values of individuality and freedom of choice encouraged in the west, were developed and owned by a middle- and upper-class elite. No doubt, in cultures where the family has always been the primary social unit, the necessity for staying together as a group to improve chances of survival was a factor in the development of strong family ties. In the west greater wealth has meant more and more individuals are able to survive as individuals and in smaller family units. Perhaps partly as a result of this it has been noticeable to me that working-class families have a much more family- and community-orientated culture than middle-class ones in this country (the UK). I see this as one of the great strengths of 'working-class culture'.

As I have rediscovered notions of parenting that are more ancient and long standing than the current professional ones, I have become less and less wedded to the professional ideas concerning normal and dysfunctional parenting that I have been taught. In my experience child and family services are often dominated by conversations about good and bad parenting with plenty of parent blaming present. Many parents find the advice they get from professionals concerning the nuts and bolts of parenting can be quite helpful. However, in my experience there are a number of pitfalls, particularly with those who hold on to the professional idea of parenting with religious intensity. If, clinically, you become too highly focused on the nuts and bolts of parenting (with the attendant professional values underpinning this) you can become worse than the overly critical, interfering grandparent that many of us professionals are taught to criticize. Going down that path can mean missing the big picture. It can mean missing many important aspects such as understanding the intentions of a parent. For example, not talking about a traumatic event or a family secret is likely to be criticized within a western, mental-health framework. If you go too quickly down this pathway you may miss the opportunity to understand that what motivates such a stance, may be the wish to protect the well-being of a loved child. Whilst the overall aim of an intervention may be similar in both cases, understanding, accepting and positively valuing the intention of the parent is likely to lead to a very different experience for that parent and a working engagement that could make all the difference to the intervention.

Keeping account of the full context is also important in keeping hold of the big picture. For example, it may be tempting to criticize a depressed mother who feels like giving up, or maybe even has given up, on parenting her children, only to discover that she has an unsympathetic husband who does not come to sessions, who goes out drinking with his friends, plays little part in child care and further criticizes his wife's attempts to parent her children. Naturally, in such a situation the critical remarks should be reserved for the unhelpful partner.

Jade was 14 years old when I first met her. She was admitted to hospital after a fit which, investigations revealed, had no physical cause. Jade had not been attending school for several months. Her parents had separated a year earlier. Her dad had intermittent contact and lots of broken engagements with the family since moving in with a new girlfriend. Jade's mum felt guilty, depressed and hopeless. During the sessions I kept praising Jade's mum for sticking by her children and I criticized their father for his lack of responsibility. I spoke about the father's behaviour towards Jade as being emotionally abusive and blamed him entirely for causing Jade's problems. Over the next few months Jade's health improved and she returned to school. She still loved her father, but had been able to blame him for the situation and had given up hope that she could get him to return home.

Professional notions of parenting really start coming undone when we work with families that have a more family, as opposed to individual, orientation. Here it is important to be able to accept, value and work with the sets of values and principles alien to the ones we are taught as professionals. For example, a common issue I have encountered which causes a degree of confusion in professional circles is that of adolescent autonomy for children from non-western families. This often shows itself in assessments and interventions for adolescent girls who self-harm. It is all too commonly assumed that the core problem is cultural conflict whereby the adolescent is striving for her own independence and autonomy and her family is stopping her from achieving this. In the intervention it is often assumed that what needs to be done is to help the young adolescent gain more autonomy from their family. In other words it is assumed that one should side with the western cultural attitudes in a culture-conflict situation. At its worst, and I have heard many professionals express this, rescue fantasies develop whereby it is felt that it is the professionals' duty to rescue the young adolescent from their dreadful family and culture.

Such simplistic notions hide many layers of more creative possibility. First, it should be recognized that when a young adolescent encounters a western professional she or he may assume (often correctly) that that person believes in individuality and autonomy for the adolescent. Consequently, many will engage with the professional around a version of events which will create and amplify a developing story the young adolescent has in their head about their culture, that leads them to criticize and maybe even disengage from their family's cultural heritage. At the same time it can also minimize and disengage that young person from the other issues that may well have been more important in the lead up to their difficulties. I remember seeing an adolescent, whose parents are Indian, after she had taken an overdose. The girl told me how her parents were too restrictive and did not allow her any freedom. I only discovered from other family members, and the girl herself, at a later date that she was in fact the spoilt one in the family and that the overdose had been triggered by her shame at being discovered after stealing money from her mother.

Second, it reduces the chances of engaging both family and the young person around a positive evaluation of their family's culture of origin (whose values may well be, and often are, in conflict with the dominant western ones). It also reduces the chance to positively evaluate the intentions of the parents. After successfully engaging a family of Asian origin, following an overdose from their daughter, her father told me 'The reason I didn't want you to see my daughter on her own when you first met us is because I don't trust psychiatrists. They usually want to see children on their own and ask them questions about their parents so that they can get them to say things that will split the family up'.

Family-life norms

Just as there is little to gain by pathologizing different styles of parenting, there is little to gain by pathologizing different family forms. There are different family forms both between and within different cultural groups – from extended families to single-parent families, from heterosexual partnership-based families to homosexual partnership-based families, from male-dominated families to female-dominated families. In my experience, when asked, most families are quite good at explaining what is normal for them, what is experienced as difficult, stressful and traumatic for them and what is not. Although I accept the idea of denial of painful experiences as a routine (and often needed) part of people's defence mechanisms, I am much less inclined to view a lack of reported stress at an event that a professional would regard as painful and difficult as always being due to denial. I think that for each of us our most frequent experiences become our normal against which we compare the rest of our experiences. I think as professionals we have to challenge ourselves to continuously reassess the assumptions that we hold which come from the cultural values and attitudes enshrined in our professional training. For example, although it is true to say that single-parent families are likely to struggle more, particularly given that statistically single-parent families are hugely over-represented in the most deprived sections of the population, if we then further stigmatize them by focusing on single parenthood as a problem (as opposed to, for example, an absent parent as the problem) we are only going to make the situation worse. Furthermore, the tendency of professional training to focus on what is wrong (i.e. pathologizing) means that we notice less of what is actually okay and going well.

Discipline

I think that one of the problems in our culture of children's rights and freedoms is that, as a culture, we have become very ambivalent about discipline. All too often the cultural message that we get, particularly as parents in public settings, is one that it is your sole responsibility (as opposed to a common social one) to ensure the good behaviour of your child. If you try to discipline your child in any way (but particularly through physical chastisement) this will be judged very critically and may even land you in big trouble with the social services. In many other cultures discipline is regarded as a common duty that is the property of all, i.e. all sorts of adults have the right and, indeed, duty to reprimand a child for wrongdoing, not just the immediate parents. There is a saying in Africa that 'it takes a village to raise a child'.

On the question of techniques used to achieve discipline, I think a lot of rubbish is written, without any real basis for understanding how the child experiences the discipline. For example, does the child experience immediate, on-the-spot physical punishment as being worse than time out, i.e. being removed to a different place (the professionally advised standard of punishment). In my experience both can bring on tears and upset and in some children the time out will be experienced as the worse and most upsetting punishment of the two. Furthermore, on the question of long-term consequences, is there really any evidence that physical chastisement leads to violent temperament. Furthermore, do we understand the long-term consequences of time-out procedures? I also think a lot of rubbish is written about the idea of non-reinforcement of negative behaviour, positive parenting and the avoidance of the idea of punishment. In my personal and professional life I meet many parents who have a good handle on their children's behaviour and whose children are well-behaved publicly and okay privately. In my experience many of them have a confident, matter-of-fact approach to punishment, some use smacking as part of their punishments and some don't. Too many families are terrorized by the professional representatives of the state where the message is to back off from controlling your children and, at the same time, if their children are out of control the message they get is that it is their fault as parents.

I find that a lot of my work around the issue of discipline revolves around the idea of deconstructing these cultural decrees. As a professional, being able to talk with families about punishment, about finding the bottom line, about understanding parents' intentions and not jumping down their throats or to unwarranted conclusions when I hear that physical punishment is sometimes involved, all helps towards to re-empowering some parents, who have become scared by punishment, to take the idea of punishment seriously again. The basic stance I take is to ask who is the boss at home and if it is not the parent, then to work with that parent to make sure that they become the boss. I explore with them what does and what does not work in terms of punishment and, in particular, towards finding a bottom line, a kind of ultimate line that children learn not to walk over. If you can find a bottom line that's working then, after a short time of using it you only need the threat of it for the desired outcome. Common bottom lines include being sent to the bedroom, removing all toys, stopping pocket money, not being allowed to watch TV, not being allowed to play on the computer, grounding and turning the electricity off.

It can be quite a task to re-empower parents to use ways of punishment that work for them, when they are surrounded by negative messages about discipline and the fear that they will be accused of silencing their children or, worse, of child abuse. Of course, I would not be encouraging empowerment in any situation where I considered abuse was taking place. I am also aware that if I was practising this approach in Iraq, my country of origin, thinking with parents about discipline (which is regarded as a duty for Muslim parents) would not be such a loaded cultural issue as it is in this country.

Child protection

Few of us would argue that in a modern, civilized society having safeguards in law for vulnerable and voiceless groups such as children is a necessity. Few of us would argue with the evidence that suggests those who experience child abuse suffer (often major) mental-health problems in the long term. However, my difficulty with the current child-protection framework, as it is practised in the UK, is that it is, and ultimately will remain (like psychiatry), based on cultural-value judgements, which can lead to very damaging discrimination. Furthermore, I have to wonder how much a child-protection framework has become a necessity as a result of our culture developing in a way that is, at its heart, quite child unfriendly. For example, has the greater sexual liberalism in our society meant that we are less able to protect our children from negative consequences of a more sexually stimulated society? It remains a serious question to me whether actual physical sexual abuse has increased as a result of this constant over-stimulation of our sexual imagination. I expect it has. In addition, the world is a potential playground for the rich, western countries. For many survival means money, in these circumstances it is hardly surprising that the trend for developing all sorts of routes to sexual satisfaction (including paedophilia) is spreading, with the result that children all over the world are terribly exploited.

My point in mentioning all of this is that before we get too heavy and judgemental on other countries' records of treating their children, we should take a little time to consider the appalling and damaging record of our own culture in the way it treats and protects children.

I have encountered a particular problem with the issue of physical abuse in many families where well-intentioned parents have found themselves in trouble. One particular group where the child-protection culture of this country comes as a shock and surprise, is refugee families. Refugee families often come into this country after difficult and complex circumstances in their own. Without knowledge of the child-protection system in this country, families carry on practising discipline in the manner they have been used to. Typically a child who has been physically chastised at home then hears that this is not acceptable in this country and in his or her immediate upset state tells a teacher. Social services are informed and a child-protection investigation ensues. Although no further action may be taken, the family is warned not to use any further physical chastisement and a complete reversal of the normal power relationship within the household then occurs. The parents back off, feeling humiliated, and the child begins to assume more control. As the child learns of their many rights within our culture, they may even threaten to contact teachers, social services or the police if their parents do not do as they wish. Family relationships break down, the child becomes out of parental control and the mental-health consequences are disastrous for all. The older the child the more difficult it is to reverse this dynamic once it has been put in motion by a child-protection investigation.

The question of emotional abuse and neglect is much harder to pin down. Within the four categories of child abuse used in this country – sexual abuse, physical abuse, emotional abuse and neglect – it is only the first two that are clearly based on concrete physical events that have occurred to the child. Yet, the thing that may be the most damaging to any child's long-term mental health is the mental torture that may result, for example, from chronic rejection, scapegoating and lack of positive attention. I feel that it is these more qualitative judgements that, by their nature, are more difficult, need more experience and more training, that are lacking in the way the child-protection framework is practised in this country. For example, a father who shows little attention towards and then abandons his children (as very often happens in this individualist, libertarian culture) can cause awful mental-health consequences for that rejected child. However, if the father had stuck around and given that child a smack every now and then, he is more likely to be accused of child abuse than the abandoning father, who has probably caused more damage. How can this be right? It is an absolutely absurd situation and highlights the cultural distortion of the child-protection framework.

When asked to work with and see families where the child-protection framework has become involved, our role is often to try and understand the qualitative aspects of the situation. We try to understand something about the emotions, the level of connection between people and the intentions of those accused of abuse. For some parents, who were perhaps over-vigorously trying to discipline their child, it might mean acting as an advocate on their behalf. At the same time I believe the child-protection framework needs to be continuously challenged. I have, on more than one occasion, tried to get social services to become involved in a child-protection investigation where a child was, in my opinion, suffering serious mental-health problems as a result of qualitatively painful situations such as chronic rejection by one or both parents. The child-protection system basically functions to remove children from the abusive situation. There are many problems with this. Some children may experience being taken into care as a punishment for having spoken out about the situation at home, the result being that they lose, not just the abusive person, but their home and family. Furthermore, for many children the care system itself exposes them to even more abuse and rejection. In contrast, parents who are guilty of rejection or abandonment, are left unpunished by the law.

Schools and education

When visiting schools and observing classes, you soon discover that standards and techniques vary from school to school, class to class, teacher to teacher, one time of day to another, and so on. Just as with different family forms there are, I am sure, many different successful teaching methods, and just as different family forms produce different sorts of issues and problems, so do different teaching methods. The primary thrust of teaching methods these days seems to be towards a teaching style that encourages the development of self-responsibility and works on motivation for learning (as opposed to somebody telling you what to do all the time). There are many teaching environments. In Iraq (where I grew up) the classes had rows of desks with one point at the front for the child to focus on, this was the blackboard at the front of the room where the teacher stood. Going around schools in the UK today, I cannot help comparing the environments children learn in, with those in which I grew up. In the schools I visit I am likely to see children sitting in groups around tables, working on projects with the teacher wandering around between tables. The physical environment is often of a highly stimulating nature full of coloured posters, pictures, with books in one corner, toys in another, a computer in another, various things hanging from the ceiling and so on. It has always struck me that these environments are a lot more interesting and enjoyable looking than the teaching environments I grew up with, but they are also more difficult to patrol and control with far more distractions. Perhaps this has something to do with why boys in particular seem to do less well in this sort of 'difficult to contain' environment. Perhaps the fact that the vast majority of them are taught by a female teacher, who may find it easier to relate to girls, may also contribute to a further discrimination against boys. For many families who come to the clinics I have worked in, a central concern is school based, be it behavioural or academic. Many have come as result of pressure from their child's school. Some hope that as a psychiatrist I may be able to put my finger on just what disorder it is that has caused the problems. Getting into schools, observing a classroom, talking to teachers, arranging meetings for teachers and parents, reviewing expectations, finding out about bullying policies, finding out about what extra resources a class needs to deal with certain children, finding out about their special educational needs section, and emotional and behavioural support, looking at patterns of referrals from particular schools, discovering certain interests of particular schools, speaking with head teachers, advocating for certain parents, developing homework routines, in other words getting engaged with school as a big part of the child's life is invaluable in helping many children and families. All too often schools are hoping that an outside agency is the key to changing a child's behaviour. All too often schools are stretched with their resources, under pressure from performance league tables and school inspections and may feel relieved to have a child 'calmed down' using medication. All too often my role is to get the school involved in getting their 'hands dirty', examining what they themselves could do, as opposed to passing the problem on to someone else.

Verbal and non-verbal communication

In the western-developed therapies the emphasis is consistently on verbal communication as the higher order communication used to resolve difficulties. Psychoanalytic psychotherapy, cognitive therapy, family therapy, indeed the whole idea of psychological sophistication is based on the ability to communicate verbally. There is a hierarchical thread within western professional culture implying that the more articulate you are, the greater your psychological sophistication and the less articulate you are, the more primitive and backward you are. This is not the case in all cultures, particularly where a mind–body split has not become as dominant as it has in western culture.

It stands to reason that in a more lived-emotion-centred culture (as opposed to articulated-emotion-centred culture), states of distress will often be expressed through the body (psychosomatic). Whether one way of being distressed is superior to another is, in my view, open to question.

Similarly, it is in my view open to question whether a therapist who relies on articulated emotion is superior to the one who uses lived emotion. My personal experience has been that the more comfortable I have become with living my emotions in my work (as opposed to distancing myself from emotional contact with clients) the more helpful and effective my clients have experienced me to be. These days I feel happier to use instinct, intuition and my emotions more actively and less reflectively. Using non-verbal communication such as coming to the child's house or school, playing with a child, sending a personal letter, full involvement in the greeting and goodbye rituals, the way you shake hands, touching someone sympathetically on the shoulder, expressing shock, surprise, anger, pain, becoming bored, telling somebody off, praising them to the sky and so on, all helps model a more relaxed, flexible way of relating which I think sends clients important messages at a non-verbal level.

I am also much more interested in the idea of developing balances, for example looking at diets, routines, exercise, stimulation, relaxation, sleeping patterns, nurture and discipline, and so on. Sometimes I have found this approach, i.e. providing a frame to get an out-of-balance life back into balance, a useful and effective alternative to medication in a number of common problems, for example with naughty boys and with depression.

Gender issues

Gender seems to have passed us by completely in child psychiatry. Yet the gender distribution could not be starker. It requires some thought even if there is no apparent interest within the profession in engaging with this issue. In most child-psychiatric departments three to four times more boys are referred than girls. The most common psychiatric diagnoses of childhood are three or more times more commonly diagnosed in boys than girls. We don't see many fathers in our routine clinical work, most of it taking place with mothers (I have often wondered whether there was a link between the fact that we see mainly boys and very few fathers, in fact I have often wondered if a child-psychiatry department functions a bit like a surrogate father in a culture where fathers appear to be opting out of parenting without any other back-up system, such as a well-functioning extended family, being in place). Academic theories are full of mother blaming and a focus on the mother/child relationship with little mention of fathers (although recently a few authors have finally started paying serious attention to fathers and fatherhood). Staff ratios in the majority of institutions dealing with young children (such as primary schools and child-psychiatry departments) tend to be female dominated. Then there is also the issue of stereotyping men from developing countries as being sexist and oppressive to women and children. I expect there are many more examples of gender issues such as the above. Why aren't we, as a profession, discussing them?

I often try hard to involve uninvolved fathers by first working towards finding a way to get them to attend (perhaps sending a personal letter of invitation or phoning them up). Where possible I like to talk with them about father/son things, man-to-man chats, differences between boys and girls, male role models and about things boys like to do with their fathers. Where a father has clearly opted out of his duty and responsibility then I will join the mother in criticizing that father, often in front of the child. In such a situation I am trying to direct the anger and hurt a child feels, towards the right target, to reduce self blame and to model a different sort of male father attitude. Sometimes I meet mothers who are struggling to control their son's behaviour but who, on closer questioning, don't have a model in their mind of how to deal with boys (e.g. they only had sisters, or their parents had not loved them for whatever reason). In such situations I like to chat about how boys' behaviour can be different to girls', to re-look at what their expectations are of their sons and to open up conversations around what you have to do to gain control of boys' as opposed to girls' behaviour.

John, an only child, was 7 years old when I first met him. He was hyperactive at home, never listened and his school complained that he had poor concentration. His father worked away for many weeks then would be home for many weeks. On average he was away from home for about 6 months a year. After a couple of sessions with John and his mother, I asked about John and his father's relationship in more detail. His mum revealed that his father finds it very difficult to spend any time with John, feeling that John rejects him. She couldn't remember the last time

John and his father had done anything together. I wrote to John's father inviting him to meet me and followed this up with a brief telephone call. On meeting him he confirmed how difficult he found it relating to John. I discussed with him the importance of a father, particularly to a son, and suggested that he start building up this relationship by doing things together, just the two of them, regularly. I suggested that, as with many things in life, the more you put in, the more you'll get out. I never saw him again but carried on meeting with John and his mother. She told me of the big change that had happened in John's relationship with his dad and John spoke about his dad quite frequently in the sessions thereafter. His behaviour, pretty much from that moment, calmed down and he was discharged.

Supernatural explanations and possession states

It is important to understand that, if you have lived and experienced the world around you in terms of supernatural explanations, then these explanations must be taken seriously, respected and valued. The idea of possession by some sort of negative force is an ancient one and has some equivalents, I believe, in western, mental-health theories. For example, Michael White's externalizing of symptoms approach is very similar to a model of possession treated by exorcism. Here the client or family is viewed as separate from a problem that has gained control over them. The treatment revolves around the idea of making this problem external to the client, so that the client or family can develop strategies to fight and get rid of or get control over this externalized problem. This idea that an otherwise normal, well-functioning person comes to be possessed by a mysterious, negative force of some sort, comes up in many different versions in other western but more rationalist approaches to mental health. For example, psychoanalysts may speak of a person becoming possessed by eruptions from the unconscious, in other words that unresolved, unconscious conflicts are triggered by some event and surface as a symptom that takes possession and control of the person. Perhaps the most popular one in the current excitement about genetic explanations is the idea that genes lay dormant until a certain stage when their expression is triggered, then these mutant genes take possession of the person, resulting in behaviour that the person experiences as being outside their control. The more I have worked with possession models the more impressed I have become with possession as a basic model to frame many mental-health conditions. It is also a frame that can help develop a non-blaming approach.

It seems to me that the basic parameters for a possession is an apparently relatively normal person who then develops a condition that appears to take control of him or her to the point of changing their life and causing significant handicap. The different models above explore the idea of what has caused this possession from a different starting point. The religious healer may see this in terms of an evil, supernatural spirit. The psychoanalyst may see it in terms of unresolved, developmental conflicts. The geneticist may see it in terms of the expression of genetic material that had, until that moment, lain dormant. Most of these theoretical approaches seem to consider the affected person as being likely to have some pre-existing vulnerabilities. In addition, it is often viewed as requiring a trigger event.

Although it is sometimes helpful to start looking at and trying to understand the causes behind a possession state, my impression has been that this is best done once the person possessed is gaining the upper hand again over its possessor. Consequently, in conditions where I am taking the possession model as the basic framework, I usually start by trying to get a measure of how much the person possessed feels they still have control over their lives and how much they feel the possession has taken control over their lives. I often give the possession a name early on. For example in a child suffering with anorexia nervosa I might be asking how much the child him- or herself feels they have control over their lives and how much they feel the anorexia has taken control. I try to differentiate early on between what thoughts are being generated by the person and what thoughts are being generated by the possession. For example, in the above case every time the person thinks I must not eat this or that, I would ask if that were their thoughts or the anorexia's. Often, during a session, I may have reason to say 'hang on a minute that was the anorexia answering me, now I want to hear what you would say' and I would get the person to try, there and then, to fight the possession to gain control of their thoughts. I often have reason to 'flesh out' the possession and give it a bigger persona (e.g. I may talk about anorexia as a bully and discuss what tactics it uses to try and keep the upper hand). Within the intervention I often take the approach of setting up a team to help the young person fight the possession (e.g. the young person's parents, myself and maybe a particularly trusted friend, sibling or other relative). The basic model thereafter is one of all of us trying to take control back from the possession. Sometimes, particularly with primary-school-age children, I use diaries of this struggle, in which a score out of ten is given each day to how strong the child has been and how strong the possession has been. Sometimes I use goals and targets to help motivate and recognize change. Sometimes I role play with the young person the internal battle. For example, I will role play the possession and ask the young person to be themselves arguing back. Sometimes, particularly with younger children, I use some favourite characters of theirs to try and catch their imagination, for example, them as Superman trying to defeat the Joker (the possession). There is a lot of room for creativity in developing the battle tactics within such a frame, in a whole range of conditions such as eating disorders, depression, obsessive compulsive disorder, distressing auditory hallucinations, temper tantrums and other forms of aggression.

Working with psychosis

My personal model of working with psychosis has been developed through working with a limited number of adolescents and young adults often with a first episode of psychosis and often without the advantage of a community-team backup. My ideas and conclusions are therefore sketchy and lacking in experience. My impression has been that a mental-state examination is both unnecessary and often a hindrance to attempting to engage with the young person and understand to some degree what they may be trying to communicate. I have certainly found that the more I attempt to understand the young person presenting with psychosis (in other words presenting with symptoms and behaviours that we consider beyond the realm of our everyday understanding and that lead us to conclude that the sufferer has lost touch with reality) the less likely I am to reach a conclusion that what they are saying or doing is completely non-understandable, and the more likely I am to develop some simple human engagement with the sufferer. While there may be exaggerations, distortions and peculiarities, there is usually, in my experience, a core that makes some sense. Consequently, with a first presentation of psychosis I usually take the following approach to an intervention.

First, I try my best to avoid labelling that young person as having a major mental illness. Mental-health labels (such as schizophrenia or manic depression) not only have major stigmatizing effects, but also labelling can result in a tunnel vision in everybody's impression of that young person. I usually stick to a broad category and idea such as psychotic for an unknown reason. This way the idea is built in that this may be short lived and that, at this stage, it is possible that it will be a single episode from which the person may well recover and be perfectly healthy thereafter. Second, I try to engage the young person in whatever way I can using intuition and the feelings I get in the company of the client. I give-on-the spot comments and interpretations, even if this means plucking at straws. My aim is to develop some kind of basic contact which can be worked on and developed. Third, I try to engage the family and enquire about what explanations they have for the situation. I usually find it is possible to develop a complex framework of possible explanations from the start. Fourth, I give the family the choice of trying to manage the situation at home or referring the client to an in-patient unit. Nearly always I have found that with some discretion and offers of support, most people are keen to see if they can find a way to manage the young person in the home setting, at least initially. If they do decide on treating the young person at home then I suggest the basic framework is that of transferring the hospital ward into the home setting. The client then benefits from the familiarity and comforts of home being present. Of course in some cases it is partly the stress of the home environment that needs to be relieved and therefore transfer to an in-patient unit is indicated. If the family and client decide to stay at home, it often means discussing with the family what extra support they have, who can do what at what time and other such practical day-to-day things. It often means having a discussion about medication both with the young person and with the family. It often means continuing to try and understand and make sense of what is going on for the young person. Suggestions from all sorts of other approaches often come in (be they seeing a religious healer, applying for a course, getting a routine up and running, working on the diet, looking at past experience, etc.). It usually means a higher level of support and commitment than to most clients with, certainly in the initial stages, weekly visits and frequent telephone calls to discuss various issues with the family and so on. The basic approach is to try to make sense and find some meaning in what the psychotic client may be trying to communicate whilst developing a containing environment. Most relatives (particularly for a first presentation) can live with the idea that the person is not ill (medically) but unwell and seem glad and thankful that someone is trying to understand the predicament of their child.

Throwing out the bath water (whilst keeping the baby)

My professional trainings have not been dumped but I have felt compelled to challenge them in many ways. Perhaps the biggest change has occurred in my attitude to the beliefs and value systems I was taught in my training. They are part of my intuitive shopping bag of ideas, beliefs and techniques that have become as much a part of me as all the other rich and varied influences in my life. These different models slide in and out of consciousness during any session, experience making this as natural as riding a bicycle. The man-made boundaries between the models have slowly blurred and dissolved. I understand there is a danger that comes from a loosening of the boundaries around a framework. There is a fear that if beliefs begin to lose their strength, their potency will also be diluted. However, I have also learned that the adaptability and flexibility that such an approach offers, better reflects the post-modern complexity in which we have to conduct our business.

The following are a few notes critically reflecting on some of the valuable bits of thinking that different professional models have given me.

Psychiatry

My medical training has helped me become aware of the body and understand known physical variables. Perhaps the most important contribution is that of developing the confidence to use medication where necessary, as another tool available to me in my shopping bag of things to use. On the whole, however, I think I use medication much more sparingly than the majority of my colleagues. I often take the attitude that my role is to provide as much information as possible about medication so that a joint decision can be taken by myself and the client, about whether or not to use it. What I have not been able to feel comfortable buying into is the child-psychiatric system of diagnosis, which, to my mind, lacks objective validity. I have no difficulty in sharing with clients the process of how I would arrive at a diagnosis and, if requested, whether they (or in the case of parents, their children) satisfy the criteria for any diagnosis. I am also comfortable to share with and discuss with clients my basic problem with diagnosis, which is that it does not tell you about the cause of the difficulty, it just gives the impression that it does. Furthermore, as a framework for intervention I have found the psychiatric framework, despite its hierarchical status, rather tunnel visioned and often unhelpful. Of course the medical model has an appeal in terms of its simplicity (symptoms, diagnosis, treatment) and as a readily accessible and acceptable framework in most cultures at present (because of its colonial ambitions). However, in my experience most individuals and families are much more interested and ready to take on complexity than we give them credit for.

Psychotherapy

My psychotherapy training has, I believe, taught me a lot and influenced my clinical approach enormously. Taking a long-term perspective, tolerating not knowing, refraining from advice at times, use of and reflection on feelings generated in a session, letting human relationships unfold naturally (less human relationship engineering), looking after my own emotional state and resisting the need to fix people, are just a few of the enduring qualities I feel the psychotherapy approach has helped to develop within me.

Family therapy

Family-therapy approaches have also been very influential in developing a lot of my thinking. Family-therapy theory and practice has helped me develop my awareness that we exist in a network of relationships. This has sensitized me into not making too many rash assumptions about what the most powerful source of impact on any individual is. Individuals not only exist in families with all their powerful interrelationships, but they also go to schools, have peers, have pressures of work, need social support networks, live with or without extended families and are subject to the impact of all sorts of other social and cultural pressures from neighbours, chats, news reports, magazine articles, advertising, etc. I have also found the family-therapy literature to be, generally speaking, more interested in the impact of political realities on our lives and therefore more interested in exploring how issues such as gender, culture, race, sexuality, family forms and so on, impact on theory and practice in mental health. Surprisingly, though, class issues seem to me to have passed family therapy (as well as all the other therapies) by.

Cognitive and behavioural therapy

I must confess to never feeling very comfortable with cognitive behavioural approaches. I always felt that these were basically common-sense approaches (derived from the common knowledge, particularly of a management-orientated culture) cloaked in some scientific terms with the cheek then to call themselves a scientific therapy. I have also found the mechanical and rather impersonal nature of the prescribed way of carrying out these therapies inhibiting of creativity and not something I could easily engage with. Having said all of that, I know I am constantly using what would be regarded as behavioural and cognitive techniques. However, to my mind, I am simply using ordinary, common sense with the advantage of experience and without the formal strait-jacket of a behavioural or cognitive therapy. I use cognitive behavioural approaches therefore in a way that fits with my personality.

This chapter has basically been a brief whirlwind through some of the changes that have occurred as my mind was opened up to alternative approaches. It reflects on a personal journey through the world of therapies as the landscape of my working mind came to be populated by a more complex map. It is difficult to know these days if the core of that map is built around the one I developed through my training. But then the mind remains too mysterious for us to understand everything about it and that is the way it is likely to remain, at least in my lifetime.

Finally, just a note to say that I decided to write this chapter in this personal reflective style in a probably rather feeble attempt to get across the impression that changing and developing new approaches is part of an ordinary human process with coincidences, meeting of certain influential people, changes in life circumstances, disappointments, joys, etc. I made a conscious attempt to steer clear of a more academic, perhaps prescriptive, approach of this is how you should or shouldn't do it. I had enough of that during my training.

Chapter 9

The future of child and adolescent psychiatry

Child and adolescent psychiatry, as a relatively young profession, has the opportunity to take a developmental pathway that is different to that of general psychiatry, a pathway that doesn't repeat the mistakes made there and that engages fully with the controversies. We should be able to engage in debates about values, beliefs, politics, context and indeed the very core assumptions that dominate this field.

The dominant approach to general psychiatry has changed little in the last century. The medical model reigns supreme and the basic diagnostic categories imposed are based on those originally developed by doctors in the late nineteenth and early twentieth centuries. A colleague of mine jokingly said to me 'whilst the rest of medicine has grown and developed new modern techniques, psychiatry is still using the horse and cart'. There has been a spectacular failure to get any biological handle on the physical causes of the mental-health problems that psychiatrists deal with. Theories continue to come and go – it's an endocrine problem, it's a hormonal problem, it's to do with ion transport systems in the membrane, it's a genetic disorder, it's due to a dysfunction of the frontal lobe, the temporal lobe, the caudate nucleus, the hypothalmus, it's to do with lack of dopamine receptors, it's to do with too many dopamine receptors, it's a problem with cell migration, it's related to blood flow in the brain, it's a problem with filter mechanisms, it's a deficiency in a part of the brain to do with theory of mind, it's to do with a lack of maturation of the newer parts of the brain, it's a form of dementia, it's a form of allergic reaction, etc. If these core assumptions had been viewed and approached in a strictly scientific manner, then surely by now we would have been revisiting the basic assumptions, the basic categories and the basic way we conceptualize mental-health problems in our discipline. However, faith is a powerful emotion. It is necessary for a continued sense of existing in a meaningful way. These beliefs based on faith will therefore not shift easily or comfortably. The faithful continue to believe that enlightenment will come and that these discoveries will be made.

Because of this lack of scientific evidence, psychiatry has left itself open to many criticisms throughout the twentieth century, to which it has reacted defensively in its attempt to continually reassert its medical identity (Clare, 1976). The best-known challenge to modernist psychiatry is the so-called anti-psychiatry movement of the 1960s and 1970s (see Chapter 5). Since then challenges to orthodox, modernist psychiatry have been voiced by several different movements. The so-called 'new transcultural psychiatry' has been vocal in criticizing orthodox psychiatry for not giving proper consideration to context in the concepts it uses. This is particularly apparent when the cultural context is considered. Here it becomes evident that the psychiatric categories in use are developed from a particular cultural and philosophical history based in western enlightenment and whose shortcomings and failings become more obvious when applied to other cultures with a different history, set of beliefs and values (see, e.g. Kleinman, 1988; Littlewood and Lipsedge, 1989; Fernando, 1988).

Another important challenge to modernist psychiatry has come from the growth of user movements in the past two decades. User movements seem to have grown up out of a shared dissatisfaction and criticism of the psychiatric services. There are examples of personal accounts and experiences (Pembroke, 1991; Lindow, 1993) which concentrate on what they consider to be an abusive system. There are also instances of more widespread examination of psychiatric services from a user perspective (Van Hoorne, 1992; Campbell, 1993). There is also a large body of research demonstrating that users are not satisfied with current practice in mental-health services (Rogers *et al.*, 1993; Wood, 1994). Predictably, little has been published in the medical literature regarding this movement (Cohen, 1998), despite government policy in the UK for the past 10 or so years being that of promoting greater user involvement in all aspects of decision-making processes within mental-health services (Wedderburn-Tate, 1994, Bracken and Thomas, 2001). The user movements present many challenges to psychiatrists, which they will have to take on board. These include being able to listen critically to the voice and criticisms of the user movement, to move into a more co-operative stance with patients (as opposed to imposed, paternalistic expertise), to debate with patients and society ethical issues of psychiatric practice, to reappraise our understanding of mental illness (something which may involve partially relinquishing or re-negotiating a psychiatrist's position of power and influence) and to develop care models and treatments which are acceptable to patients (Cohen, 1998).

Another important strand of challenge to mainstream, orthodox psychiatry comes from clinicians incorporating post-modern thinking into their clinical practice. This comes at a time when faith in psychiatry, medicine, indeed science and technology as a whole, has been diminishing in the general population. With concerns about values as well as evidence, preoccupation with risk as well as benefit and the rise of the well-informed patient, medicine as a whole is having to look at and re-negotiate its relationship to the patient and society (Muir-Gray, 1999). As I have argued in this book, psychiatry faces the additional problem that its own beliefs in its modernist achievements are themselves disputed. Bracken and Thomas (2001) argue that psychiatry needs to adapt to the reality of this post-modern environment which requires a rethinking of the goals of psychiatry through giving a greater importance to contexts (social, political and cultural), to developing an ethical rather than technological orientation in our practice and to rethink the politics of coercion. Such an approach does not seek to replace the techniques (including medical ones) used in psychiatry but to democratize mental health by linking progressive service development to a debate about contexts, values and partnerships. Some of these ideas have been successfully incorporated into service delivery (e.g. Bracken and Cohen, 1999).

These various attempts to open up thinking and ideas in a way that influences practice within psychiatry has created a tension between the strong 'modernist' influences such as evidence-based medicine and these 'post-modernist' challenges (Laugharne, 1999). Evidence-based medicine is clearly a modernist idea that has been contributing to, and partially resolving some therapeutic dilemmas within mainstream medicine. Thus far it has had little impact on the theories used in psychiatry, particularly when you consider that the prevailing evidence suggests that the system of classification on which we base treatments is fundamentally unscientific. But, as has often been pointed out, even apparently scientific beliefs do not arise in isolation or are necessarily based on good evidence, as scientific discourse is itself rooted in the social community of scientists (Mathers and Rowland, 1997). Clients' own preoccupations are often at odds with those of evidence-based medicine, as what is statistically determined on a large population may be interpreted very differently by the individual patient who may conclude that 'what is right for the majority may not be right for me' (Leggett, 1997). This leaves an ongoing tension for psychiatrists between the continuing push for greater technicalization of their jobs through so-called 'evidence-based' practice and the simple human demands from our clients, of being able to listen to their own particular narratives (Greenhalgh, 1999).

Child psychiatry has yet to engage these debates. I have seen little evidence of active questioning of the central assumptions and constructs we use, on which we base research, service delivery and our interventions. This seems to me to be not only unscientific and undemocratic, but a state of play that is leading to a very ill-thought, continued, creeping, medicalization of a profession that appears to have learned little from the difficulties its older sibling, general psychiatry, has been through. We urgently need a critical debate within the profession about the fundamental concepts we use and the fundamental ideas behind the way that we organize services, influence service development and develop our interventions. We need to engage with the multicultural reality of the post-modern world. We need to humanize and detechnicalize many aspects of our practice. We need to be aware of the powerful status we are given in society and how our way of thinking about matters such as unhappiness, activity, social communication and many other behaviours in children and adolescents, influences thinking about important social matters, not only with our clients but in our culture more generally. Until the profession has shown the democratic maturity to engage with these debates, then the type of child psychiatry we are practising bears a great resemblance to pre-1960s general psychiatry, an era where the only debate occurring was sterile competition between different medically derived models for understanding the human problems we deal with.

Developing training for child and adolescent psychiatrists

If practice is going to change within child and adolescent psychiatry, then future child and adolescent psychiatrists need to be exposed to alternative models of practice and thinking. Arguably, for this to happen the climate must also have shifted within general-psychiatry training as child psychiatrists are first trained as general adult psychiatrists before training as child and adolescent psychiatrists. Although it would appear that the younger generation of psychiatrists are more interested in questions of culture and philosophy, the mainstream in the UK remains dominated by medical-model psychiatry and this is reflected in the structure and content of the professional exams for membership of the Royal College of Psychiatrists. As Fernando (1988) suggested, any strategies to free psychiatry sufficiently so that real changes can take place must seek to enlist the support of the Royal College of Psychiatrists. Although the status and power of an organization like the Royal College of Psychiatrists makes challenges leading to important changes seem futile, psychiatry, just like other branches of medicine, has had to start responding to the growing influence from user movements. In addition the debate in the UK on the effects of institutional racism has begun to impact on medical institutions as witnessed by the recent book *Racism in Medicine* (Coker, 2001). Institutional change is always slow and difficult. If this can be borne in mind then continual challenges (including books such as this) can help the gradual chipping away of the old order.

The faculty of child and adolescent psychiatry represents the sub-specialty within the Royal College of Psychiatrists. As I have attempted to show in this book, it is plagued by the same conceptual inadequacies and biases as the rest of psychiatry. Therefore, my first suggestion for developing a healthier training for child and adolescent psychiatrists is that of active resistance. This can be done on many fronts, as an individual, in groups and through service developments. A book like this is an act of resistance. Raising uncomfortable issues in a conference is an act of resistance. Challenging your trainer's unacknowledged racism is an act of resistance. Circulating an article written by a user on their experience of medication is an act of resistance. Developing a non-medical-model-based service is an act of resistance.

If child-psychiatric training is to become more progressive then the current trend towards appointing so-called neuropsychiatrists as professors in academic child and adolescent psychiatry departments must change. Having been trained on a child-psychiatric training scheme where a professor whose main interest was in neuropsychiatry organized the training, I believe I have first-hand experience of the inevitable dominance of the western medical model in this scheme. Neuropsychiatry is a peculiar western invention, a field which is inevitably culture blind and produces training schemes which are not even going to get to the starting block in terms of addressing questions relating to belief systems and culture.

In an ideal world child psychiatric training would be structured so as to reflect the relative nature of our psychiatric belief system. This could be done in several ways to reflect the central issue of the social construction of meaning. One way would be to develop a problem-solving approach to teaching. Thus, teaching sessions would revolve around taking a clinical problem, exploring what different meanings this clinical problem could have when viewed through different frameworks (including a medical one) and exploring the different possible ways of dealing with this problem as guided by different theoretical frameworks. An alternative model could be one where different theoretical frameworks are studied in some depth (e.g. a term per framework) having first laid down (perhaps during the first term) the cultural underpinnings to any system by studying the social construction of meaning. Whatever the structure used the importance of understanding how our belief systems are culturally constructed, of developing a user-centred attitude, of deconstructing the hierarchical assumptions of our profession, and of being able to question the universality of our assumptions would be vital. If we wish to develop a user-sensitive, culturally appropriate, non-racist and democratic profession, then I believe these are the sorts of changes that must happen in our training.

Changes needed in research

As I hope I have shown in this book, research published in the major academic child and adolescent psychiatry journals and textbooks uses a conceptually weak framework to interpret its findings. It uses questionnaires whose cross-cultural validity has not been established and routinely makes assumptions and draws conclusions that are, in my opinion, essentially racist, sexist and stigmatizing. There is a basic problem in the way the understandable current trend for evidence-based practice in the rest of medicine is being applied to sub-specialties like child psychiatry. The evidence base we have in child psychiatry has little to do with material physical facts about our client group and a lot to do with assumptions about what constitutes a disorder and what a desirable outcome to treatment should be.

As a result mainstream child-psychiatry research has come to rely too heavily on medical-model-inspired methods as the gold standard. Thus, the recent multicentre trial comparing Ritalin® treatment with behavioural treatment and community treatment packages for children diagnosed with so-called ADHD (MTA Co-operative Group, 1999a, 1999b) concluded that we now have a good evidence base to suggest that Ritalin® and possibly Ritalin® alone is the best treatment for children with ADHD. As I discussed in Chapter 7, this conclusion is so full of assumptions it is worrying how many child psychiatrists have accepted it at face value. I wonder what the conclusion of this study would have been if they had built the research around a conceptually different framework. For example, instead of randomizing the children into groups receiving Ritalin® treatment, behavioural treatment, etc. (in other words, adhering with religious intensity to a particular medical research style), the first session could have been an open, informative discussion with the parents about the pros and cons and controversies concerning Ritalin®. Then parents could have made the choice as to which treatment group their children went in to. Researchers would of course criticize this approach as methodologically flawed.

I would retort that the existing study was conceptually flawed. I would rather read about research that was creative enough in its design to allow room for and empower parent choice than impose, hierarchically, a particular concept. The methodology would be different, the analysis of the findings would be different and the conclusions would hopefully have room for complexity. When it came to looking at results, surely it would be more important for us to know what the parents and the children themselves thought rather than what the doctors had decided would be a good outcome. Of course a truly radical piece of research would not even start with this scientifically and cross-culturally non-valid construct of ADHD. Even if you do accept this idea then its social construct, as opposed to medical illness credentials, must be acknowledged. This is not a small point. To me a parent and child who feel much happier after a period of treatment, even though all the original behaviours that were being complained about are still present, is as important as changing the behaviour of the child. Sometimes the real progress in tackling a problem comes not through changing the child in some way but through changing the way somebody thinks about them. If you want to stick to the medical model with a child labelled with ADHD, then ADHD treatment-outcome research (in other words the effect of treatment on so-called ADHD symptoms) would seem a valid way to increase knowledge about how to deal with children with this 'disorder'. If you are prepared to consider alternative explanations for the behaviour of an ADHD-labelled child then much of the research becomes irrelevant. If you have structured parents' (and often teachers') expectations in such a way that success can only be seen in terms of changes in particular behaviours in the child, then this standard medical research would be important to refer to. If success can also mean other things (e.g. greater acceptance of a child's behaviour, a change in the way people think about a child, getting extra support at school, etc.) then reference to the evidence from this standard, gospel, medical research becomes less useful.

Research that can grapple with conceptual issues must be encouraged. Qualitative research needs to be given a higher status, as must more in-depth analysis of conceptual issues. In adult psychiatry anthropologically trained psychiatrists, such as Arthur Kleinman and Roland Littlewood, have been influential in helping to incorporate anthropological thinking into psychiatric research. Predictably their research has not only thrown light on cultural questions but also thrown into the question the scientific validity of the psychiatric constructs we use. Such anthropologically informed research is urgently needed in child and adolescent psychiatry. One possible way forward may be through collaboration with family therapists. There has been a useful debate going on within family therapy circles about the nature of childhood and the family and which has been considerably enriched by interest in ideas from sociology, politics and anthropology (e.g. Krause, 1998).

As with training, these changes are unlikely to happen without challenges to those in positions of greatest power (e.g. editorial boards of child and adolescent journals). As with training, creating a climate of challenge and resistance is necessary.

Changes needed to service delivery

We must recognize that the organizations we work for are part of the communities we live in. Not only do they provide a service for children and families but they also contribute to local, cultural belief systems about problems of children and how to deal with them. Services need to recognize the impact they have on local populations. Services should be sensitive and mindful of local needs and issues. I attend far too many management meetings in which the professionals are too busy trying to protect their own identity and professional esteem to be able to take the necessary risks to make them more accessible to users. I have been to many meetings where professionals have managed to put the brakes on developing the practice of sending a copy of our letters to the GP, to the family. The fear seems to be that users won't understand what we're talking about, so that what we write could end up unnecessarily upsetting them. Instead of seeing this as a threat to our professional relationship with clients, we should view this as a challenge to practices and attitudes that are based on suspicion and mistrust of clients.

Child and adolescent mental-health services can be made more user friendly and accessible in a number of ways. First, the issue of staffing must be considered particularly in an area where the service is based in a multicultural environment. The background of staff members in such institutions needs to reflect the multicultural background of the community it is serving. Incorporating staff from different ethnic groups brings with it many problems that need to be acknowledged by the management and tackled. During my time as a consultant in a multicultural area of London I contributed towards a service development which involved employing bilingual co-workers who spoke some of the local languages. The project was conceptualized as one in which two-way learning could occur. The bilingual co-workers, who already had experience as health advocates for the local community, would be learning some of our ideas and techniques and at the same time it was envisaged that the therapists and psychiatrists in our institution would learn from the co-workers more about the local community's values, beliefs and practices. After 18 months of establishing this project and service, the bilingual co-workers' perceptions were that the other professionals were under-utilizing them and when they did use them it was only as an interpreter. The management, whilst being very happy to get all the public relations credentials for establishing this project, found it very difficult to acknowledge this problem of, in effect, institutionalized racism. The management, once they were made aware of this problem, was, perhaps understandably, reluctant to broach this issue with the other professionals in the service. None the less, with persistence some progress was made. To me it illustrated how difficult it is to incorporate non-mainstream thinking into mainstream services. Incorporating staff from the local communities who spoke the local languages created a new cultural challenge for an institution dominated by white western frameworks and belief systems.

Second, service users' views should always be sought. This does not have to be a complicated task. It can be incorporated into all assessments, either informally through the practitioner's routine clinical practice or formally through question-naires, through use of suggestion boxes or through formal research conducted by those who are not members of the treatment service.

Third, and perhaps most importantly, is our being able, as clinicians, to develop an attitude of curiosity in other people's beliefs, together with an ability to question our assumptions. I discuss how this impacts on clinical work in Chapters 6 and 8.

Fourth, child and adolescent psychiatry departments need to be able to offer a range of treatment approaches if they are to be considered holistic. To me holistic treatment does not mean a multidisciplinary carving up of a child and their family's problems, in fact it is the opposite. A situation where the doctor is seeing a family to review medication, a social worker is doing some parent training with the parent, and a therapist is seeing the child for individual therapy is not necessarily an example of holistic medicine. Often this solution complicates life for the child and their family far more than is necessary. Holistic skills are something that services should encourage in individual practitioners. A holistic approach means individual practitioners having the ability to work with the whole picture, to use multiple frameworks and understand different perspectives. When more than one professional is involved they are, as far as possible, not working at cross purposes and as if the other's work is irrelevant to what they are doing. Holistic services should also be able to make use of the voluntary sector, where sometimes you are more likely to find local, culturally appropriate and knowledgeable services that have been developed by members of the local community. In areas where the local community uses traditional healing practices and complimentary medicine then a project that incorporates these practices (e.g. through employment of complimentary and traditional practitioners or formal systems of consultation with such practitioners) should be established.

Some examples

Although the task of challenging mainstream child and adolescent psychiatry to shift in a more progressive direction seems overwhelming it is certainly not impossible. There are examples from existing practice, where both training and service delivery have been influenced to develop towards the multi-framework approach I have been advocating in this book.

The tri-cultural organization of the New Zealand 'Just Therapy' group (Tamasese and Waldegrave, 1993) developed after a period of consultation between a family centre in New Zealand and representatives of the local Maori and Polynesian Island communities. Through the development of a dialogue, therapists in the family centre began to question the appropriateness of the concepts they used, particularly when it came to working with indigenous Maori and Polynesian communities. This eventually led to the introduction of three sections in their organization – a white western section, a Maori section and a Pacific Island section. Each section worked predominantly with clients from the community they represented and were staffed by members from that community. The 'Just Therapy' group developed ideas that became so influential in New Zealand that eventually they affected statutory agencies as well as government policy. The most well-known influence of this group is the concept of family group conferences where members of the extended family are brought together to try to discuss and resolve issues around the care of children who have either been put on the 'at risk' register (for child abuse) or are being considered for this.

At the Marlborough family service in London an ongoing debate about the appropriateness of the Euro-centric approach of services, culminated in the development of a more effective training course and, eventually, a service development (Miller and Thomas, 1994; Krause and Miller, 1995). The Marlborough family service helped develop a movement for improving training in cultural issues, particularly in family therapy. On a service-delivery level this led to the development of the Marlborough Asian family counselling service. Members of staff who spoke the local languages of the area were recruited and trained to become therapists able to conduct family therapy in the indigenous language of the family.

Fernando (1996) has written about a personal example of how to show resistance and challenge institutional dominance. In his article he shows how individuals who show polite irreverence for 'prized rituals and myths' of institutions can initiate change. He also noted that as a member of a non-dominant group he might be able to initiate change through this route but is always at risk of victimization.

It is always a difficult balancing act how much to challenge and how much to stay quiet, and just as Fernando found polite irreverence helped to initiate change so I have found that quiet persistence can help the process of 'chipping away'. In establishing the non-medical-model ADHD clinic that I described in Chapter 7, I met with a lot of resistance from the clinic hierarchy. As I described in Chapter 5, initially the clinic management rejected the proposal. However, rather than watering down the proposal and allowing the clinic to become just another standard 'yes, he has it/no, he does not' type clinic, I had to persist over a period of several months. After a few battles behind the scenes and some rewording of the proposal the clinic was established with the promise that we would be allowed to develop it as we wished. This we did. Quiet persistence and a resistant frame of mind were needed.

The culture and family I grew up in was built on resistance. Resistance is in my bones.

> I think it is a mistake to think of colonialism as a one-way street . . . as something so powerful you can't resist it. There is always resistance somewhere that comes out of your own culture, your language, your religion.
>
> (Sivanandan, 1990: 3)

In moments when a young child tells of the taunts at school and their family say 'ignore them they are ignorant', or, 'if he says it again hit him': resistance is forming; when an Indian parent points to a famous historical building and remarks 'even the stone – the very fabric – they stole from us', or when a

Caribbean parent says as they walk on early industrial streets that 'these streets were built on our crops': resistance is forming; when slavery or the colonization of exotic lands is re-told after school in its brutal context, or in the tension brought home from work or from public places, or in the eyes of elders when authorities knock on the door: resistance is in the making.

(Dhruev, 1992: 83)

Bibliography

Achenbach, T.M. and Edelbrock, C.S. (1978) The classification of child psychopathology: a review and analysis of empirical efforts. *Psychological Bulletin* 85: 1275–1301.

Akhmedzhanov, M. and Lifshits, A.M. (1971) On the discussion of the disease concept. *Archives of Pathology* 33: 87–90.

Aleksakhina, R. (1968) The concept of 'essence' and the question of the essence of disease. *Journal of the Academy of Medical Science* 23: 30–34.

American Psychiatric Association (1966) *Diagnostic Statistical Manual of Mental Disorders* second edition (DSM-II). Washington, DC: American Psychiatric Association.

American Psychiatric Association (1980) *Diagnostic and Statistical Manual of Mental Disorders* third edition (DSM-III). Washington, DC: American Psychiatric Association.

American Psychiatric Association (1987) *Diagnostic and Statistical Manual of Mental Disorders* third edition revised (DSM-III-R). Washington, DC: American Psychiatric Association.

American Psychiatric Association (1994) *Diagnostic and Statistical Manual of Mental Disorders* fourth edition (DSM-IV). Washington, DC: American Psychiatric Association.

Ammar, H. (1973) *Growing Up in an Egyptian Village*. New York: Octagon.

Anderson, W.T. (1990) *Reality Isn't What it Used to Be*. San Francisco: Harper & Row.

Arac, J. (1989) *Critical Genealogies: Historical Situations for Post Modern Literary Studies*. New York: Colombia University Press.

Argyle, M. (1982) 'Inter-cultural communication' in S. Bochner (ed.) *Cultures in Contact: Studies in Cross-cultural Interaction*. Oxford: Pergammon.

Babayan, E. (1985) *The Structure of Psychiatry in the Soviet Union* trans. V. Brobos and B. Meerovich. New York: International University Press.

Baldwin, S. and Anderson, R. (2000) The cult of methylphenidate: clinical update. *Critical Public Health* 10: 81–86.

Baldwin, S. and Cooper, P. (2000) How should ADHD be treated? *The Psychologist* 13: 598–602.

Bang, S. (1987) *We come as a friend*. Derby: Refugee Action.

Barkley, R. (1994) *Attention Deficit Hyperactivity Disorder*. Presentation at the Royal Society of Medicine London, 1994.

Barkley, R.A., McMurray, M.B., Edelbrock, C.S. and Robbins, K. (1990) Side-effects of methylphenidate in children with attention deficit hyperactivity disorder: a systematic, placebo-controlled evaluation. *Paediatrics* 86: 184–192.

Barnes, D.M. (1987) Biological issues in schizophrenia. *Science* 235: 430–433.

Bateson, G. (1973) *Steps to an Ecology of the Mind*. St Albans: Paladin.

Bateson, G. (1979) *Mind and Nature, a Necessary Unity*. London: Fontana.

Battle, E.S. and Lacey, B. (1972) A context for hyperactivity in children over time. *Child Development* 43: 757–773.

Baumgaertel, A., Wolraich, M.L. and Dietrich, M. (1995) Comparison of diagnostic criteria for attention deficit disorders in a German elementary school sample. *Journal of the American Academy for Child and Adolescent Psychiatry* 34: 629–638.

Bean, P., Bingley, W., Bynoe, I., Rasseby, E. and Rogers, A. (1991) *Out of Harm's Way*. London: MIND.

Bean, R. B. (1906) Some racial peculiarities of the Negro brain. *American Journal of Anatomy* 5: 353–415.

Bebbington, P.E. (1978) The epidemiology of depressive disorder. *Culture, Medicine and Psychiatry* 2: 297–341.

Bebbington, P.E. (1997) 'Social and transcultural psychiatry' in R. Murray, P. Hill and P. McGuffin (eds) *The Essentials of Postgraduate Psychiatry* third edition. Cambridge: Cambridge University Press.

Bebbington, P.E., Hurry, J. and Tennant, C. (1981) Psychiatric disorders in selected immigrant groups in Camberwell. *Social Psychiatry* 16: 43–51.

Berger, M. (1994) 'Psychological tests and assessment' in M. Rutter, E. Taylor, and L. Hersov (eds) *Child and Adolescent Psychiatry, Modern Approaches* third edition. Oxford: Blackwell Scientific Publications.

Berger, P.L and Luckman, T. (1967) *The Social Construction of Reality*. New York: Doubleday.

Berrios, G.E and Morley, S.J. (1984) Koro-like symptom in a non Chinese subject. *British Journal of Psychiatry* 145: 331–334.

Berry, J.W. (1994) 'Acculturation and psychological adaptation: an overview' in A. M. Bouvy, V. Vande, F. Vijver, P. Bowski, and P. Schmitz (eds) *Journeys into Cross-cultural Psychology*, Lisse: Swets & Zeitlinger.

Bhaskar, R. (1989) *Reclaiming Reality*. London: Verso.

Bhugra, D., Leff, J. and Mallet, R. (1977) Incidence and outcome of schizophrenia in whites, African Caribbean's and Asian's in London. *Psychological Medicine* 27: 791–798.

Biederman, J., Newcorn, J. and Sprich, S. (1991) Comorbidity of attention deficit disorder with conduct, depressive, anxiety and other disorders. *American Journal of Psychiatry* 148: 564–577.

Black, D. (1993) 'A brief history of child and adolescent psychiatry' in D. Black and D. Cottrell (eds) *Seminars in Child and Adolescent Psychiatry*. London: Gaskell.

Bloch, S. and Chodoff, P. (1991) *Psychiatric Ethics* second edition. Oxford: Oxford University Press.

Bloch, S. and Reddaway, P. (1977) *Russia's Political Hospitals*. London: Gollancz.

Bograd, M. (1984) Family systems approach to wife battering: a feminist critique. *American Journal of Orthopsychiatry* 54: 558–568.

Bombar, M.L. (1996) Putting biological approaches in context. *ISSPR Bulletin* 12: 3–6.

Boorse, C. (1975) On the distinction between disease and illness. *Philosophy and Public Affairs* 5: 49–68.

Bouhdiba, A. (1977) 'The child and the mother in Arab-Muslim society' in L.C. Brown and N. Itzkowitz (eds) *Psychological Dimensions of Near Eastern Studies*. Princeton: Darwin.

Bowlby, J. (1969) *Attachment and Loss, Volume 1, Attachment*. London: Hogarth Press.

Bowlby, J. (1973) *Attachment and Loss, Volume 2. Separation*. London: Hogarth Press.

Boyden, J. (1990) 'Childhood and the policy makers: a comparative perspective on the globalization of childhood' in A. James and A. Prout (eds) *Constructing and Reconstructing Childhood*. London: Falmer Press.

Boyle, M.H. and Jadad, A.R. (1999) Lessons from large trials: the MTA study as a model for evaluating the treatment of childhood psychiatric disorder. *Canadian Journal of Psychiatry* 44: 991–998.

Bracken, P. and Cohen, B. (1999) Home treatment in Bradford. *Psychiatric Bulletin* 23: 349–352.

Bracken, P. and Thomas, P. (2001) Post psychiatry: a new direction for mental health. *British Medical Journal* 322: 724–727.

Bradley, C. (1937) The behaviour of children receiving Benzedrine. *American Journal of Psychiatry* 94: 577–585.

Bradely, C. and Weisner, T.S. (1997) 'Introduction: crisis in the African family' in T.S. Weisner, C. Bradley and P.L. Kilbride (eds) *African Families and the Crisis of Social Change*. Westport: Bergin and Garvey.

Bradshaw, J. (1990) *Child Poverty and Deprivation in the United Kingdom*. London: National Children's Bureau.

Breggin, P.R. (1994) *The War Against Children: How the Drugs Programmes and Ttheories of the Psychiatric Establishment are Threatening America's Children with a Medical 'Cure' for Violence*. New York: St Martin's Press.

Breggin, P.R. (1997) *Brain Disabling Treatments in Psychiatry: Drugs, Electro-shock and the Role of the FDA*. New York: Springer.

Breggin, P.R. (1998) *Talking Back to Ritalin: What Doctors aren't Telling You About Stimulants for Children*. Monroe, ME: Common Courage Press.

Breggin, P.R. (1999) Psychostimulants in the treatment of children diagnosed with ADHD. Part 1 – acute risks and psychological effects. *Ethical Human Sciences and Services* 1: 13–33.

Breggin, P.R. (2000) The NIMH multimodal study of treatment for attention deficit/ hyperactivity disorder: a critical analysis. *International Journal of Risk and Safety in Medicine* 13: 15–22.

British Medical Journal News (1995) *British Medical Journal* 310: 1429.

British Psychological Society (1996) *Attention Deficit Hyperactivity Disorder (ADHD): a Psychological Response to an Evolving Concept*. Report of a working party of the BPS, London: British Psychological Society.

Bronfenbrenner, U. (1970) *Two Worlds of Childhood: USA and USSR*. New York: Russell Sage.

Brown, G. and Harris, T. (1978) *The Social Origins of Depression: a Study of Psychiatric Disorder in Women*. London: Tavistock.

Browne, D. (1990) *Black People, Mental Health and the Courts*. London: NACRO.

Burleigh, M. (1994) *Death and Deliverance: Euthanasia in Germany 1900–1945*. Cambridge: Cambridge University Press.

Buunk, B. and Hupka, R.B. (1986) Autonomy in close relationships: a cross-cultural study. *Family Perspective* 20: 209–221.

Byrne, D. and Kelley, K. (1992) Differential age preferences: the need to test evolutionary versus alternative conceptualisations. *Behavioural and Brain Sciences* 15: 96.

Campbell, M., Cohen, I.L. and Small, A.M. (1982) Drugs in aggressive behaviour. *Journal of the American Academy of Child and Adolescent Psychiatry* 21: 107–117.

Campbell, P. (1993) Mental health services – the users view. *British Medical Journal* 306: 848–850.

Cantwell, D.P. (1972) Psychiatric illness in the families of hyperactive children. *Archives of General Psychiatry* 27: 414–417.

Cantwell, D.P. (1975) 'Genetic studies of hyperactive children: psychiatric illness in biologic and adopting parents' in R. Fieve, D. Rosenthal and H. Brill (eds) *Genetic Research in Psychiatry*. Baltimore: John Hopkins University Press.

Cantwell, D. and Rutter, M. (1994) 'Classification in child and adolescent psychiatry' in M. Rutter, E. Taylor and L. Hersov (eds) *Child and Adolescent Psychiatry, Modern Approaches* third edition. Oxford: Blackwell Scientific Publications.

Cantwell, N. (1989) 'A tool for the implementation of the UN convention' in R. Barnen (ed.) *Making Reality of Children's Right*. International Conference on the Rights of the Child, New York.

Carluccio, C., Sours, J. A. and Kolb, C. (1964) Psychodynamics of echo reactions. *Archives of General Psychiatry* 10: 623–629.

Caron, C. and Rutter, M. (1991) Comorbidity in child psychopathology: concepts, issues and research strategies. *Journal of Child Psychology and Psychiatry* 32: 1063–1080.

Carothers, J.C. (1951) Frontal lobe function and the African. *Journal of Mental Science* 97: 12–48.

Carstairs, G.M. (1957) *The Twice Born*. London: Hogarth.

Castel, R. (1976) *L' Ordre Psychiatrique* trans. W. Halls, *The Regulation of Madness*. London: Polity Press, 1988.

Cecchin, G. (1987) Hypothesizing, circularity and neutrality revisited: an invitation to curiosity. *Family Process* 26: 405–413.

Cha, J.H. (1994) 'Aspects of individualism and collectivism in Korea' in U. Kim, H.C. Triandis, C. Kagitcibasi, S.C. Choi and G. Yoon (eds) *Individualism and Collectivism: Theory, Method and Applications*. Thousand Oaks: Sage.

Chakraborty, A. and Sandel, B. (1984) Somatic complaint syndrome in India. *Psychiatry Research Review* 21: 212–216.

Chapman, J. (1966) The early symptoms of schizophrenia. *British Journal of Psychiatry* 112: 225–251.

Charles, L. and Schain, R. (1981) A four year follow up study of the effects of methylphenidate on the behaviour and academic achievement of hyperactive children. *Journal of Abnormal Child Psychology* 9: 495–505.

Children's Defence Fund (1994) *The State of America's Children Yearbook: 1994*. Washington DC: Children's Defence Fund.

Chiu, T. L., Tong, J.L. and Schmidt, K.E. (1972) A clinical and survey study of Latah in Sarawak, Malaysia. *Psychological Medicine* 2: 155–165.

Christie, D., Lieper, A.D., Chessells, J.M. and Vergha-Khadem, F. (1995) Intellectual performance after presymptomatic cranial radiotherapy for leukaemia: effects of age and sex. *Archives of Disease in Childhood* 73: 136–140.

Chu, G.C. (1985) 'The emergence of a new Chinese culture' in W. Tseng and D. Wu (eds) *Chinese Culture and Mental Health*. New York: Academic Press.

Clare, A. (1976) *Psychiatry in dissent: Controversial Issues in Thought and Practice*. London: Tavistock.

Clare, A. (1997) 'The disease concept in psychiatry' in P. Murray, P. Hill and P. McGuffin (eds) *The Essentials of Postgraduate Psychiatry* third edition. Cambridge: Cambridge University Press.

Cohen, M. (1998) Users movement and the challenge to psychiatrists. *Psychiatric Bulletin* 22: 155–157.

Cohen, P., Cohen, J. and Kasen, S. (1993) An epidemiological study of disorders in late childhood and adolescence. I. Age and gender-specific prevalence. *Journal of Child Psychology and Psychiatry* 34: 851–877.

Coid, J., Kahtan, N., Gault, S. and Jarman, B. (2000) Ethnic differences in admissions to secure forensic psychiatric services. *British Journal of Psychiatry* 177: 241–247.

Coker, N. (ed.) (2001) *Racism in Medicine: an Agenda for Change*. London: Kings Fund.

Cope, R. (1989) The compulsory detention of Afro-Carribbean's under the Mental Health Act. *New Community* 15: 343–356.

Copeland, L., Wolraich, M., Lindgren, S., Milich, R. and Woolson, R. (1987) Paediatricians' reported practices in the assessment and treatment of attention deficit disorders. *Journal of Developmental and Behavioural Paediatrics* 8: 191–197.

Cramond, B. (1994) Attention deficit hyperactivity disorder and creativity: what is the connection? *Journal of Creative Behaviour* 28: 193–210.

Cunningham, H. (1995) *Children and Childhood in Western Society since 1500*. London: Longman.

Cunningham, L., Cadoret, R., Loftus, R. and Edwards, J.E. (1975) Studies of adoptees from psychiatrically disturbed biological parents. *British Journal of Psychiatry* 126: 534–539.

Currer, C. (1986) 'Concepts of mental and ill being: the case of Pathan mothers in Britain' in C. Currer and M. Stacey (eds) *Concepts of Health, Illness and Disease: a Comparative Perspective*. Lemington Spa: Berg.

Cushman, P. (1995) *Constructing the Self, Constructing America*. Reading, MA: Addison-Wesley.

Davis, S.S. and Davis, D.A. (1989) *Adolescence in a Moroccan Town*. New Brunswick, NJ: Rutgers University Press.

Davydovskii, I. (1962) *Problems of Causality in Medicine*. Moscow: The State Medical Publisher.

Davydovskii, I. and Sil-Vestrov, V. (1966) On the definition of the disease concept. *Archives of Pathology* 28: 3–8.

Dean, G., Walsh, D., Downing, H. and Shelley, P. (1981) First admissions of native born and immigrants to psychiatric hospitals in south east England, 1976. *British Journal of Psychiatry* 139: 506–512.

Delal, F.N. (1993) Race and racism: an attempt to organise difference. *Group Analysis* 26: 277–293.

Dell, P. (1982) *Pathology: the Original Sin*. Paper presented at the First International Conference on Epistemology, Psychotherapy and Psychopathology: Houston.

Dhruev, N. (1992) Conflict and race in social work practice. *Journal of Social Work Practice* 6: 77–86.

Doerner, K. (1969) *Burger und Irre. Zur Sozialgeschichte und Wissenschaftssoziologie der Psychiatrie* trans. J. Neugroschel and J. Steinberg *Madman and the Bourgeoisie: a Social History of Insanity and Psychiatry*. Oxford: Basil Blackwell, 1981.

Donnelly, M. and Rapoport, J.L. (1985) 'Attention deficit disorders' in J.M. Weiner (ed.) *Diagnosis and Psychopharmacology of Childhood and Adolescent Disorders*. New York: Wiley.

Douglas, M. (1970a) *Natural Symbols*. London: Barrie and Rockliffe.

Douglas, M. (1970b) The healing rite. *Man* 5: 302–308.

Douglas, M. (1982) 'Introduction to grid/group analysis' in M. Douglas (ed.) *Essays in the Sociology of Perception*. London: Routledge and Kegan Paul.

Douglas, V.I. (1972) Stop, look and listen: the problems of sustained attention and impulse control in hyperactive and normal children. *Canadian Journal of Behavioural Science* 4: 254–282.

Douglas, V.I. (1983) 'Attention and cognitive problems' in M. Rutter (ed.) *Developmental Neuropsychiatry*. New York: Guilford Press.

Dow, J. (1986) Universal aspects of symbolic healing: a theoretical synthesis. *American Anthropologist* 88: 56–69.

Draeger, S., Prior, M. and Sanson, A. (1986) Visual and auditory attention performance in hyperactive children: competence or compliance. *Journal of Abnormal Child Psychology* 14: 411–424.

Drug Enforcement Administration (1994) *ARCOS (Automation of Reports and Consolidated Orders Systems) Data Base 1981–1992*. Washington, DC: US Department of Justice.

Dunham, H.W. (1964) Social class and schizophrenia. *American Journal of Ortho-psychiatry* 34: 634–646.

Dwivedi, K.N. (1993a) 'Child abuse and hatred' in V.P. Varma (ed.) *How and Why Children Hate* London: Jessica Kingsley.

Dwivedi, K.N. (1993b) 'Coping with unhappy children from ethnic minorities' in V.P. Varma (ed.) *Coping with Unhappy Children*. London: Cassell.

Dwivedi, K.N. (1995a) 'Stress in children from ethnic minorities' in V.P. Varma (ed.) *Coping with Stress in Children*. Aldershot: Arena Publishing.

Dwivedi, K.N. (1995b) 'Race and the child's perspective' in G. Upton, R. Davie and V.P. Varma (eds) *The Voice of the Child: a Handbook for Professionals*. London: Falmer Press.

Dwivedi, K.N. (1996) 'Culture and Personality' in K.N. Dwivedi and V.P. Varma (eds) *Meeting the Needs of Ethnic Minority Children*. London: Jessica Kingsley.

Dwivedi, K.N. (1997) 'Management of anger and some Eastern stories' in K.N. Dwivedi (ed.) *Therapeutic Use of Stories*. London: Routledge.

Eaves, L.J., Silberg, J.L., Hewitt, J.K. *et al*. (1993) 'Genes, personality and psychopathology. A latent class analysis of liability to symptoms of attention deficit hyperactivity disorder in twins' in R. Plomin and G.E. McClearn (eds) *Nature, Nurture and psychology*. Washington, DC: American Psychological Association.

Eisenberg, L. and Kleinman, A. (1981) *The Relevance of Social Science for Medicine*. Dordrecht: D. Reidel.

Ellis, G.J. and Petersen, L.R. (1992) Socialisation values and parental control techniques: a cross-cultural analysis of child rearing. *Journal of Comparative Family Studies* 23: 39–54.

Fanon, F. (1967) *Black Skins White Masks*. London: Pluto Press.

Fergusson, D.M. and Horwood, L.J. (1993) The structure, stability and correlations of the trait components of conduct disorder, attention deficit disorder and anxiety withdrawal reports. *Journal of Child Psychology and Psychiatry* 34: 749–766.

Fergusson, D.M., Horwood, L.J. and Lloyd, M. (1991) Confirmatory factor models of attention deficit and conduct disorder. *Journal of Child Psychology and Psychiatry* 32: 257–74.

Fernando, S. (1988) *Race and Culture in Psychiatry*. London: Croom Helm.

Fernando, S. (1995) 'Social realities and mental health' in S. Fernando (ed.) *Mental Health in a Multi-ethnic Society*. London: Routledge.

Fernando, S. (1996) Black people working in white institutions: lessons from personal experience. *Human Systems* 7: 143–145.

Foucault, M. (1961) *Histoire de la folie a l'age classique*. Paris: Plon.

Foucault, M. (1965) *Madness and Civilisation. A History of Insanity in the Age of Reason*. New York: Random House.

Freedman, J. and Combs, G. (1996) *Narrative Therapy: the Social Construction of Preferred Realities*. New York: Norton.

Freud, S. (1913) *Totem and Taboo* trans. J. Strachey. London: Routledge and Kegan Paul, 1950.

Freud, S. (1927) *The Future of an Illusion*, trans. J. Strachey, London: Penguin, 1985.

Freud, S. (1930) 'Civilisation and its discontents' in *Civilisation, Society and Religion*. London: Penguin, 1985.

Frieden, N. (1981) *Russian Physicians in the Era of Reform and Revolution, 1856–1905*. Princeton: Princeton University Press.

Fulford, K., Smirnov, A. and Snow, E. (1993) Concepts of disease and the abuse of psychiatry in the USSR. *British Journal of Psychiatry* 162: 801–810.

Furman, E. (1974) *A Child's Parent Dies: Studies in Childhood Bereavement*. New Haven, CT: Yale University Press.

Furman, R. (1996) Methylphenidate and 'ADHD' in Europe and the U.S.A. *Child Analysis* 7: 132–145.

Fyfe, A. (1989) *Child Labour*. Cambridge: Polity Press.

Gadow, K.D. (1983) Effects of stimulant drugs on academic performances in hyperactivity and learning disabled children. *Journal of Learning Disabilities* 16: 290–299.

Gallucci, F., Bird, H.R., Berardi, C., Galli, V., Pfanner, P. and Weinberg, A. (1993) Symptoms of attention deficit hyperactivity disorder in an Italian school sample: findings of a pilot study. *Journal of the American Academy of Child and Adolescent Psychiatry* 32: 1051–1058.

Garber, S.W., Garber, M.D. and Spizman, R.F. (1996) *Beyond Ritalin*. New York: Harper Perennial.

Gelder, H., Gath, D. and Mayou, R. (eds) (1989) *The Oxford Textbook of Psychiatry* second edition. Oxford: Oxford University Press.

Gergen, K.J., Gulerce, A., Lock, A. and Misra, G. (1996) Psychological sciences in cultural context. *American Psychologist* 51: 496–501.

Gilles de la Tourette, G. (1885) Étude sur une affection nerveuse caractérisée par de l'incoordination mortrice, accompagnée d'écholalie et de coprolalie. *Archives de Neurologie* 9: 19–42.

Gilligan, C. (1982) *In a Different Voice*. Cambridge, MA: Harvard University Press.

Gillis, J.J., Gilger, J.W., Pennington, B.F. and DeFries, J.C. (1992) Attention deficit disorder in reading-disabled twins: evidence for genetic etiology. *Journal of Abnormal Child Psychology* 20: 303–315.

Giroux, H. (1983) *Theory and Resistance in Education: a Pedagogy for the Opposition*. London: Heinemann.

Glaser, D. (1993) 'Emotional abuse' in C. Hobbs and J. Wynne (eds) *Bailliere's Clinical Paediatrics*. London: Ballier Tindall.

Glick, C.B. (1967) Medicine as an ethnographic category: the Gimi of the New Guinea highlands. *Ethnology* 6: 31–56.

Goffman, E. (1961) *Asylums*. New York: Anchor.

Goldner, V. (1985) Feminism and family therapy. *Family Process* 24: 31–47.

Goldner, V. (1988) Generation and gender: normative and covert hierarchies. *Family Process* 27: 17–31.

Goodman, R. (1997) An over extended remit. *British Medical Journal* 314: 813–814.

Goodman, R. and Stevenson, J. (1989) A twin study of hyperactivity. II: The aetiological role of genes, family relationships and perinatal adversity. *Journal of Child Psychology and Psychiatry* 30: 691–709.

Gorell-Barnes, G. (1994) 'Family Therapy' in M. Rutter, E. Taylor and L. Hersov (eds) *Child and Adolescent Psychiatry, Modern Approaches* third edition. Oxford: Blackwell Scientific Publications.

Graham, P. (1976) Management in child psychiatry: recent trends. *British Journal of Psychiatry* 129: 97–108.

Graham, P. (1986) *Child Psychiatry – a Developmental Approach*. Oxford: Oxford University Press.

Graham, P. and Stevenson, J. (1985) A twin study of genetic influences on behavioural deviance. *Journal of the American Academy of Child and Adolescent Psychiatry* 24: 33–41.

Green, C. and Chee, K. (1997) *Understanding ADHD: a Parent's Guide to Attention Deficit Hyperactivity Disorder in Children*. London: Vermilion.

Greenhalgh, T. (1999) Narrative based medicine in an evidence based world. *British Medical Journal* 318: 323–325.

Greenhill, L. (1998) 'Childhood ADHD: pharmacological treatments' in P. Nathan and J. Gorman (eds) *A Guide to Treatments that Work*. Oxford: Oxford University Press.

Greenwood, J.D. (1994) *Realism, Identity and Emotion: Reclaiming Social Psychology*. London: Sage.

Griffith, J.L. and Griffith, M.E. (1994) *The Body Speaks: Therapeutic Dialogues for Mind–Body Problems*. New York: Basic Books.

Gupta, S.S. (1970) *A Study of Women in Bengal*. Calcutta: Indian Publications.

Hall, G.S. (1904) *Adolescence: its Psychology and its Relationship to Physiology, Anthropology, Sociology, Sex, Crime, Religion and Education* vol. II. New York: D. Appleton.

Hardham, V. (1996) 'Embedded and embodied in the therapeutic relationship: understanding the therapist's use of self systemically' in C. Flask and A. Perlesz (eds) *The Therapeutic Relationship in Systemic Therapy*. London: Karnac Books.

Hardyment, C. (1995) *Perfect Parents: Baby-care Advice Past and Present*. Oxford: Oxford University Press.

Hare-Mustin, R.T. (1978) A feminist approach to family therapy. *Family Process* 17: 181–194.

Hare-Mustin, R.T. (1987) The problem of gender in family therapy theory. *Family Process* 26: 15–28.

Harvey, D. (1989) *The Condition of Postmodernity*. Manchester: Blackwell.

Hazell, P. (1997) The overlap of attention deficit hyperactivity disorder with other common mental disorders. *Journal of Paediatric Child Health* 33: 131–137.

Heath, D.T. (1995) 'Parents socialisation of children' in B.B. Ingoldsby and S. Smith (eds) *Families in Multicultural Perspective*. New York: Guilford Press.

Heelas, P. and Lock, A. (1981) *Indigenous Psychologies: the Anthropology of the Self*. London: Academic Press.

Hendrick, H. (1994) *Child Welfare England 1870–1989*. London: Routledge.

Hendrick, H. (1997) 'Constructions and reconstructions of British childhood: An interpretive survey, 1800 to the present' in A. James and A. Prout (eds) *Constructing and Reconstructing Childhood: Contemporary Issues in the Sociological Study of Childhood*. London: Falmer Press.

Hetchman, L., Weis, G. and Perlman, T. (1984) Young adult outcome of hyperactive children who received long-term stimulant medication. *Journal of the American Academy of Child and Adolescent Psychiatry* 23: 261–269.

Heyman, R. (1994) Methylphenidate (Ritalin): newest drug of abuse in schools. *Ohio Paediatrics* spring: 17–18.

Hill, G.N. 'An essay on the prevention and cure of insanity', quoted in A. Scull (1979) *Museums of Madness*. London: Allen Lane.

Hill, P. and Cameron, M. (1999) Recognising hyperactivity: a guide for the cautious clinician. *Child Psychology and Psychiatry* 4: 50–60.

Hindmarsh, H.J. (1993) Alternative family therapy discourses: it is time to reflect (critically). *Journal of Feminist Family Therapy* 5: 2–28.

Hinshaw, S.P. (1987) On the distinction between attention deficits/hyperactivity and conduct problems/aggression in child psychopathology. *Psychological Bulletin* 101: 443–463.

Hinshaw, S.P. (1994) *Attention Deficit Disorders and Hyperactivity in Children*. Thousand Oak, CA: Sage.

Hodes, M. (1998) Refugee children may need a lot of psychiatric help. *British Medical Journal* 316: 793–794.

Hoffman, L. (1991) A reflexive stance for family therapy. *Journal of Strategic and Systemic Therapies* 10: 4–17.

Hofstede, G. (1980) *Cultures Consequences: International Differences in Work-related Values*, Beverley Hills: Sage.

Hofstede, G. (1983) 'Dimensions of national cultures in fifty cultures and three regions' in J.B. Deregowski, S. Dziurawiec and R.C. Annis (eds) *Expiscations in cross-cultural psychology*. Lisse: Swets & Zweitlinger.

Hofstede, G. (1994a) 'Forward' in U. Kim, H.C. Triandis, C. Kagitcibasi, S.C. Choi and G. Yoon (eds) *Individualism and Collectivism; Theory, Method and Applications*. Thousand Oaks: Sage.

Hofstede, G. (1994b) *Cultures and Organisations: Software of the Mind*. London: HarperCollins.

Homans, G.C. (1993) 'Behaviourism and after' in A. Giddens and J. Turner (eds) *Social Theory Today*. Cambridge: Polity Press.

Horton, R. (1967) African traditional thought and Western science. *Africa* 37: 50–71.

Hsu, F.L. (1983) *Rugged Individualism Reconsidered*. Knoxville: University of Tennessee Press.

Hsu, J. (1985) 'The Chinese family: relations, problems and therapy' in W. Tseng and D. Wu (eds) *Chinese Culture and Mental Health*. New York: Academic Press.

Humphries, S. (1981) *Hooligans or Rebels? An Oral History of Working Class Childhood and Youth, 1889–1939*. Oxford: Blackwell.

Humphries, S., Mack, J. and Perks, R. (1988) *A Century of Childhood*. London: Sidgwick & Jackson.

Hunter, R. and Macalpine, I. (1963) *Three Hundred Years of Psychiatry*. London: Oxford University Press.

Huynh, H., Luk, S.L., Singh, R., Pavaluri, M. and Mathai, J. (1999) Medium-term outcome of children given stimulants for attention deficit hyperactivity disorder. *Child Psychology and Psychiatry Review* 4: 610–617.

Hynd, G.W. and Hooper, S.R. (1995) *Neurological Basis of Childhood Psychopathology*. London: Sage Publications.

Inden, R.B. (1990) *Imagining India*. Cambridge, MA: Basil Blackwell.

Jackson, S. (1985) 'Acedia, the sins and its relationship to sorrow and meloncholia' in A. Kleinman and B. Good (eds) *Culture and Depression*. Berkley: University of California Press.

Jahoda, G. (1990) 'Our forgotten ancestors' in J. Berman (ed.) *Nebraska Symposium on Motivation, 1989*. Lincoln: University of Nebraska Press.

James, A. and Prout, A. (eds) (1990) *Constructing and Reconstructing Childhood: Contemporary Issues in the Sociological Study of Childhood*. London: Falmer Press.

Janzen, J. (1978) *he Quest for Therapy in Lower Zaire*. Berkeley: University of California Press.

Jellinek, M. (1999) Changes in the practice of child and adolescent psychiatry: are our patients better served? *Journal of the American Academy of Child and Adolescent Psychiatry* 38: 115–117.

Jenhs, C. (1996) *Childhood*. London: Routledge.

Jensen, A.R. (1969) How much can we boost IQ and scholastic achievement? *Harvard Educational Review* 39: 1–123.

Johnstone, L. (2000) *Users and Abusers of Psychiatry* second edition. London: Routledge.

Jones, E. (1995) 'The construction of gender in family therapy' in C. Burck and B. Speed (eds) *Gender, Power and Relationships*. London: Routledge.

Jung, C.G. (1930) Your Negroid and Indian behaviour. *Forum* 83: 193–199.

Kagitcibasi, C. (1982) Old age security value of children: cross-national socio-economic evidence. *Journal of Cross-cultural Psychology* 13: 29–42.

Kagitcibasi, C. (1991) Decreasing infant mortality as a global demographic change: a challenge to psychology. *International Journal of Psychology* 26: 649–664.

Kagitcibasi, C. (1996) *Family and Human Development across Cultures. A View from the Other Side*. Hove: Lawrence Erlbaum.

Kakar, S. (1978) *The Inner World: a Psychoanalytic Study of Childhood and Society in India*. Delhi: Oxford University Press.

Kakar, S. (1982) *Shamans, Mystics and Doctors: a Psychological Inquiry into India and its Healing Traditions*. New York: Knopf.

Kamsler, A. (1990) 'Her story in the making: therapy with women who were sexually abused in childhood' in C. White and M. Durrant (eds) *Ideas for Therapy with Sexual Abuse*. Adelaide: Dulwich Centre Publications.

Kardiner, A. and Ovesey, L. (1951) *The Mark of Oppression. A Psychosocial Study of the American Negro*. New York: Norton.

Karon, B.P. (1994) Problems of psychotherapy under managed care. *Psychotherapy in Private Practice* 2: 55–63.

Keeney, B.P. (1983) *Aesthetics of Change*. New York: Guilford Press.

Kendall, R. (1975) The concept of disease and its implications for psychiatry. *British Journal of Psychiatry* 127: 305–315.

Kenny, M.G. (1978) Latah, the symbolism of a putative mental disorder. *Culture, Medicine and Psychiatry* 2: 209–301.

Kewley, G.D. (1998) 'Attention deficit hyperactivity disorder is under-diagnosed and under-treated in Britain. *British Medical Journal* 316: 1594–1595.

Kewley, G.D. (1999) The relevance of ADHD for paediatricians. *BACCH News* summer: 18–21.

Kiev, A. (1968) *Psychiatry in the Communist World*. New York: Science House.

Kim, U. (1994) 'Significance of paternalism and communalism in the occupational welfare system of Korean firms: a national survey' in U. Kim, H.C. Triandis, C. Kagitcibasi, S.C. Choi and G. Yoon (eds) *Individualism and Collectivism: Theory, Method and Applications*. Thousand Oaks: Sage.

King, A. and Bond, M. (1985) 'The confucian paradigm of man: a sociological view' in W. Tseng and D. Wu (eds) *Chinese Culture and Mental Health*. New York: Academic Press.

Kirmayer, L. (1984) Culture, affection and somatization, parts 1 and 2. *Transcultural Psychiatry Research Review* 21: 159–188, 237–262.

Klein, D.N. and Riso, L.P. (1994) 'Psychiatric disorders: problems of boundaries and comorbidity' in C.G. Costello (ed.) *Basic Issues in Psychopathology*. New York: Guilford Press.

Klein, R.G. and Mannuzza, S. (1991) Long-term outcome of hyperactive children: a review. *Journal of the American Academy of Child and Adolescent Psychiatry* 30: 383–387.

Kleinman, A. (1977) Depression, somatization and the new cross-cultural psychiatry. *Social Science and Medicine* 11: 3–10.

Kleinman, A. (1987) Anthropology and Psychiatry. The role of culture in cross cultural research on illness. *British Journal of Psychiatry* 151: 447–454.

Kleinman, A. (1988) *Rethinking Psychiatry: from Cultural Category to Personal Experience*. New York: The Free Press.

Kleinman, A. (1996) China: the epidemiology of mental illness. *British Journal of Psychiatry* 169: 129–130.

Kleinman, A. and Good, B. (1985) 'Introduction: culture and depression' in A. Kleinman and B. Good (eds) *Culture and Depression*. Berkley: University of California Press.

Kleinman, A. and Song, L.H. (1979) Why do indigenous practitioners successfully heal: a follow-up study of indigenous practice in Taiwan. *Social Science and Medicine* 130: 7–26.

Kohn, A. (1989) Suffer the restless children. *Atlantic Monthly* November: 90–100.

Kohn, M.L. (1987) Cross-national research as an analytic strategy. *American Sociological Review* 52: 713–731.

Kohn, M.L., Naoi, A., Schoenbach, C., Schooler, C. and Slomczynski, K.M. (1990) Position in the class structure and psychological functioning in the United States, Japan and Poland. *American Journal of Sociology* 95: 964–1008.

Kolvin, I. (1973) 'Evaluation of psychiatric services for children in England and Wales' in J.K. Wing and J. Hafner (eds) *Roots of Evaluation*. Oxford: Oxford University Press.

Kopelman, L. (1990) On the evaluative nature of competency and capacity judgements. *International Journal of Law and Psychiatry* 13: 309–329.

Kraeplin, E. (1913) *Manic Depressive Insanity and Paranoia* trans. R.M. Barclay, of *Lehrbuch der Psychiatrie* vol. 3 and 4. Edinburgh: Livingstone.

Kraeplin, E. (1920) 'Die Erscheinungs formen des Irreseins' trans. H. Marshall, in S. Hirsch and M. Shepherd (eds) (1974) *Themes and Variations in European Psychiatry. An Anthology*. Bristol: John Wright.

Kraeplin, E. (1962) *One Hundred Years of Psychiatry*. London: Peter Owen.

Krause, I. (1989) Sinking heart: a Punjabi communication of distress. *Social Science and Medicine* 29: 563–575.

Krause, I. (1998) *Therapy across Culture*. London: Sage.

Krause, I. and Miller, A.C. (1995) 'Culture and family therapy' in S. Fernando (ed.) *Mental Health in a Multi-ethnic Society*. London: Routledge.

Kumar, K.T. (1992) To children with love. *British Medical Journal* 305: 1582–1583.

Kutchins, H. and Kirk, S. (1999) *Making us Crazy. DSM: The Psychiatric Bible and the Creation of Mental Disorders*. London: Constable.

Lahey, B.B., Applegate, B., McBurnett, K. and Biederman, J. (1994) DSM-IV field trials for attention deficit hyperactivity disorder in children and adolescents. *American Journal of Psychiatry* 151: 1673–1658.

Laing, R.D. (1960) *The Divided Self*. London: Tavistock.

Lambo, A. (1969) 'Traditional African cultures and Western medicine' in F.N.L. Poynter (ed.) *Medicine and Culture*. London: Wellcome Institute of the History of Medicine.

Langford, J. (1995) Ayurvedic interiors: Person, space and episteme in three medical practices. *Cultural Anthropology* 10: 330–366.

Lasch, C. (1980) *The Culture of Narcissism*. London: Norton (Abacus).

Lau, A. (1996) 'Family therapy and ethnic minorities' in K.N. Dwivedi and V.P. Varma (eds) *Meeting the Needs of Ethnic Minority Children*. London: Jessica Kingsley.

Laugharne, R. (1999) Evidence based medicine, user involvement and the post modern paradigm. *Psychiatric Bulletin* 23: 641–643.

Laungani, P. (1992) Cultural variations in the understanding and treatment of psychiatric disorders: India and England. *Counselling Psychology Quarterly* 5: 231–224.

Law, I. (1997) 'Attention deficit disorder – therapy with a shoddily built construct' in C. Smith and D. Nyland (eds) *Narrative Therapies with Children and Adolescents*. New York: Guilford Press.

Leff, J. (1973) Culture and the differentiation of emotional states. *British Journal of Psychiatry* 123: 299–306.

Leff, J. (1981) *Psychiatry Around the Globe*. London: Gaskell.

Leggett, J. (1997) Medical Scientism: good practice or fatal error. *Journal of the Royal Society of Medicine* 90: 97–101.

Lewis, A. (1967) *The State of Psychiatry*. London: Routledge and Kegan Paul.

Liberman, J.A. and Koreen, A.R. (1993) Neurochemistry and neuroendocrinology in schizophrenia: a selective review. *Schizophrenia Bulletin* 19: 371–429.

Lieberman, A.F. and Pawl, J.H. (1990) 'Disorders of attachment and secure base behaviour in the second year of life' in M.T. Greenberg, D. Cicchetti and E.M. Cummings (eds) *Attachment in the Preschool Years*. Chicago: University of Chicago Press.

Lindgren, S., Wolraich, M., Stromquist, A., Davis, C., Milich, R. and Watson, D. (1994) *Re-examining Attention Deficit Disorder*. Paper presented at the 8th Annual Meeting of the Society for Behavioural Paediatrics: Denver.

Lindow, V. (1993) Survivor, activist or witch. *Asylum* 7: 5–7.

Littlewood, R. (1986) 'Russian dolls and Chinese boxes: an anthropological approach to implicit models of comparative psychiatry' in J. L. Cox (ed.) *Transcultural Psychiatry*. London: Croom Helm.

Littlewood, R. (1995) Psychopathology and personal agency: modernity, culture change and eating disorders in South Asian societies. *British Journal of Medical Psychology* 68: 45–63.

Littlewood, R. (1999) Roland Littlewood in conversation with Rosalind Ramsey. *Psychiatric Bulletin* 23: 733–739.

Littlewood, R. and Lipsedge, M. (1989) *Aliens and Alienists*. London: Unwin Hyman Ltd.

Livingston, R. (1999) Cultural issues in the diagnosis and treatment of Attention Deficit Hyperactivity Disorder. *Journal of the American Academy of Child and Adolescent Psychiatry* 38: 1591–1594.

Long, N. (1996) Parenting in the USA: growing adveristy. *Clinical Child Psychology and Psychiatry* 1: 496–483.

Lowe, R. (1991) Post modern themes and therapeutic practices: notes towards the definition of family therapy. *Dulwich Centre Newsletter* 3: 41–52.

Luk, S.L. and Leung, P.W.L. (1989) Connors teachers rating scale – a validity study in Hong Kong. *Journal of Child Psychology and Psychiatry* 30: 785–794.

Luke, S. (1974) *Power: A Radical View*. London: Macmillan.

Lutz, L. (1985) 'Depression and the translation of emotional words' in A. Kleinman and B. Good (eds) *Culture and Depression*. Berkley: University of California Press.

Lyotard, J.F. (1986) *The Postmodern Condition: a Report on Knowledge*. Manchester: Manchester University Press.

McCarty, C., Weisz, J., Wanitromanee, K. *et al.* (1999) Culture, coping and context: primary and secondary control among Thai and American youth. *Journal of Child Psychology and Psychiatry* 40: 809–818.

McGee, R., Feehan, M. and Williams, S. (1990) DSM III disorders in a large sample of adolescents. *Journal of the American Academy of Child and Adolescent Psychiatry* 29: 611–619.

McGee, R., Feehan, M., Williams, S. and Anderson, J. (1992) DSM-III disorders from age 11 to age 15 years. *Journal of the American Academy for Child and Adolescent Psychiatry* 31: 50–59.

McGinnis, J. (1997) Attention Deficit Disaster. *The Wall Street Journal* 18 September.

McGuiness, D. (1989) 'Attention deficit disorder, the Emperor's new clothes, Animal "Pharm" and other fiction' in S. Fisher and R. Greenberg (eds) *The Limits of Biological Treatments for Psychological Distress: Comparisons with Psychotherapy and Placebo*. Hillsdale, NJ: Lawrence Erlbaum Associates.

McKinnon, L. and Miller, D. (1987) The new epistemology and the Milan approach: feminist and socio-political considerations. *Journal of Marital and Family Therapy* 13: 139–155.

Mann, E.M., Ikeda, Y., Mueller, C.W. *et al.* (1992) Cross-cultural differences in rating hyperactive-disruptive behaviours in children. *American Journal of Psychiatry* 149: 1539–1542.

Mares, P., Henley, A. and Baxter, C. (1985) *Healthcare in Multicultural Britain*. Cambridge: Health Education Council and National Extension College.

Maslow, A.H. (1987) *Motivation and Personality* third edition. New York: Harper & Row.

Massey, I. (1991) *More than Skin Deep: Developing Anti-racist Multicultural Education in Schools*. London: Hodder Stoughton.

Mathers, N. and Rowland, S. (1997) General practice – a postmodern speciality. *British Journal of General Practice* 47: 177–179.

May, M. (1973) Innocence and experience in the evolution of the concept of juvenile delinquency in the mid-nineteenth century. *Victorian Studies* 17: 7–29.

May, R. (2000) Psychosis and recovery. *Open Mind* 106: 24–25.

Mayr, E. (1981) *The Growth of Biological Thought*. Cambridge, MA: Harvard University Press.

Meredith, W.H. and Abbott, D.A. (1995) 'Chinese families in later life' in B.B. Ingoldsby and S. Smith (eds) *Families in Multicultural Perspective*. New York: Guilford Press.

Merrow, J. (1995) ADHD – a dubious diagnosis. *Public Broadcasting Service (USA)* 5 November.

Merskey, H. and Shafran, B. (1986) Political hazards in the diagnosis of sluggish schizophrenia. *British Journal of Psychiatry* 148: 247–256.

Messing, S. (1968) Interdigitation of mystical and physical healing in Ethiopia. *Behavioral Science Notes* 3: 87–104.

Meyer, J.E. (1998) The fate of the mentally ill in Germany during the Third Reich. *Psychological Medicine* 18: 575–581.

Miatra, B. and Miller, A. (1996) 'Children, families and therapists: clinical considerations and ethnic minority cultures' in K.N. Dwivedi and V.P.Varma (eds) *Meeting the Needs of Ethnic Minority Children*. London: Jessica Kingsley.

Miller, A. and Thomas, L. (1994) 'Introducing ideas about racism and culture into family therapy training. *Context* 20: 25–29.

Miller, S., Hubble, M. and Duncan, B. (1995) No more bells and whistles: effective therapy doesn't have much to do with either theory or technique. *Family Therapy Networker* 19: 53–63.

Miringoff, M. (1994) *Monitoring the Social Well-being of the Nation: the Index of Social Health*. Tarytown, NY: Fordham Institute for Social Policy.

Mitchell, T. (1988) *Colonising Egypt*. Berkley: University of California Press.

Mitskevich, S. (1969) *Notes of a Physician Activist*. Moscow: The State Medical Publisher.

Moerman, D. (1979) Anthropology of symbolic healing. *Current Anthropology* 20: 59–80.

Monk, G., Winslade, J., Crocket, K. and Epston, D. (eds) (1997) *Narrative Therapy in Practice: the Archaeology of Hope*. San Francisco: Jossey-Bass.

Mrazek, D. (1994) 'Psychiatric aspects of somatic disease and disorders' in M. Rutter, E. Taylor and L. Hersov (eds) *Child and Adolescent Psychiatry, Mmodern Approaches* third edition. Oxford: Blackwell Scientific Publications.

MTA Co-operative Group (1999a) A 14-month randomized clinical trial of treatment strategies for attention deficit/hyperactivity disorder. *Archives of General Psychiatry* 56: 1073–1086.

MTA Co-operative Group (1999b) Moderators and mediators of treatment response for children with attention deficit/hyperactivity disorder. *Archives of General Psychiatry* 56: 1086–1096.

Muir-Gray, J.A. (1999) Postmodern medicine. *Lancet* 354: 1550–1553.

Murphy-Berman, V., Levesque, H.L. and Berman, J.J. (1996) UN convention on the rights of the child. *American Psychologist* 51: 1257–1261.

Murray, R. (1997) 'Schizophrenia' in R. Murray, P. Hill and P. McGuffin (eds) *The Essentials of Postgraduate Psychiatry* third edition. Cambridge: Cambridge University Press.

Murray, R., Hill, P. and McGuffin, P. (eds) (1997) *The Essentials of Postgraduate Psychiatry* third edition. Cambridge: Cambridge University Press.

Nandi, D.N. (1980) Socioeconomic status and mental morbidity in certain tribes and castes in India. *British Journal of Psychiatry* 136: 73–85.

Nash, J. (1967) The logic of behaviour: curing in a Maya Indian town. *Human Organization* 26: 132–140.

National Institutes of Health (1998) *Consensus Statement: Diagnosis and Treatment of Attention Deficit Hyperactivity Disorders*. Rockville, MD: National Institute of Mental Health.

Neimeyer, R. and Mahoney, M. (eds) (1995) *Constructivism in Psychotherapy*. Washington DC: American Psychological Association.

Obeyesekere, G. (1977) The theory and practice of psychological medicine in Ayurvedic tradition. *Culture, Medicine and Psychiatry* 1: 155–181.

Obeyesekere, G. (1985) 'Depression, Buddhism and the work of culture in Sri Lanka' in A. Kleinman and B.J. Good (eds) *Culture and Depression*. Berkley: University of California Press.

Offord, D.R., Boyle, M. and Szatmari, P. (1987) Ontario child health study: II. six-month prevalence of disorder and rates of service utilization. *Archives of General Psychiatry* 44: 832–836.

Offord, E. (1998) Wrestling with the whirlwind: an approach to the understanding of ADD/ADHD. *Journal of Child Psychotherapy* 24: 253–266.

Orlick, T., Zhou, Q.Y. and Partington, J. (1990) Co-operation and conflict within Chinese and Canadian kindergarten settings. *Canadian Journal of Behavioural Science* 22: 20–25.

Pare, D.A. (1996) Culture and meaning: expanding the metaphorical repertoire of family therapy. *Family Process* 35: 21–42.

Parker, I., Georgaea, E., Harper, D., McLaughlin, T. and Stowell-Smith, M. (1995) *Deconstructing Psychopathology*. Thousand Oaks: Sage.

Parry, A. and Doon, R. (1994) *Story Re-visions: Narrative Therapy in the Postmodern World*. New York: Guilford Press.

Parre, D. (1995) Of families and other cultures: the shifting paradigm of family therapy. *Family Process* 34: 1–20.

Pearson, G. (1983) *Hooligan: A History of Respectable Fears*. London: MacMillan.

Pembroke, L. (1991) Surviving psychiatry. *Nursing Times* 87: 30–32.

Perry, B.D., Pollard, R.A., Blackeley, T.L., Baker, W.L. and Vigilante, D. (1995) Childhood trauma, the neurobiology of adaptation and the use-dependent development of the brain, how states become traits. *Infant Mental Health Journal* 16: 20–33.

Pilgrim, D. (1997) *Psychotherapy and Society*. London: Sage.

Pilgrim, D. and Rogers, A. (1994) Something old, something new: sociology and the organisation of psychiatry. *Sociology* 28: 521–538.

Pincus, H.A., Tanielian, T.L. and Marcus, S.C. (1998) Prescribing trends in psychotropic medications. *Journal of the American Medical Association* 279: 526–531.

Postman, N. (1983) *The Disappearance of Childhood*. London: W.H. Allen.

Prendergast, M., Taylor, E., Rapoport, J.L. *et al*. (1988) The diagnosis of childhood hyperactivity: a US–UK cross-national study of DSM-III and ICD-9. *Journal of Child Psychology and Psychiatry* 29: 289–300.

Prince, R. and Tcheng-Laroche, F. (1987) Culture bound syndromes and international disease classifications. *Culture, Medicine and Psychiatry* 11: 3–19.

Prior, M. and Sanson, A. (1986) Attention deficit disorder with hyperactivity: a critique. *Journal of Child Psychology and Psychiatry* 27: 307–319.

Rapoport, J.L., Buchsbaum, M.S., Zahn, T., Weingartner, H., Ludlow, C. and Mickkelsen, E.J. (1978) Dextroamphetamine: cognitive and behavioural effects in normal prepubertal boys. *Science* 199: 560–563.

Rapoport, J.L., Buchsbaum, M.S., Zahn, T., Weingarten, H., Ludlow, C. and Mickkelsen, E.J. (1980) Dextroamphetamine: its cognitive and behavioural effect in normal and hyperactive boys and normal men. *Archives of General Psychiatry* 37: 933–943.

Rappley, M.D., Gardiner, J.C., Jetton, J.R. and Howang, R.T. (1995) The use of methylphenidate in Michigan. *Archives of Paediatric and Adolescent Medicine* 149: 675–679.

Rapport, M.D. (1995) 'Attention deficit hyperactivity disorder' in M. Hersen and R.T. Ammerman (eds) *Advances in Abnormal Child Psychology.* Hillsdale, NJ: Lawrence Erlbaum Associates.

Rhee, S.H., Waldman, I.D., Hay, D.A. and Levy, F. (1995) Sex differences in genetic and environmental influences on DSM-III-R attention deficit hyperactivity disorder (ADHD). *Behaviour Genetics* 25: 285.

Rie, H., Rie, E., Stewart, S. and Anbuel, J. (1976) Effects of Ritalin on underachieving children: a replication. *American Journal of Orthopsychiatry* 45: 313–332.

Riley, D. (1983) *War in the Nursery: Theories of the Child and Mother.* London: Virago.

Robin, A.L. and Barkley, R.A. (1998) *ADHD in Adolescents: Diagnosis and Treatment.* New York: Guilford Press.

Rogers, A., Pilgrim, D. and Lacey, R. (1993) *Experiencing Psychiatry: Users Views of Services.* London: Macmillan.

Rogoff, B. and Chavajay, P. (1995) What's become of research on the cultural basis of cognitive development? *American Psychologist* 50: 859–877.

Roland, A. (1980) Psychoanalytic perspectives on personality development in India. *International Review of Psychoanalysis* 1: 73–87.

Rose, N. (1985) *The Psychological Complex: Psychology, Politics and Society in England 1869–1939.* London: Routledge & Kegan Paul.

Rose, N. (1990) *Governing the Soul: the Shaping of the Private Self.* London: Routledge.

Rose, S. (1998) Neuro genetic determinism and the new euphenics. *British Medical Journal* 317: 1707–1708.

Rosenberg, C. (1975) 'The crises of psychiatric legitimacy: reflection on psychiatry medicine and public policy' in G. Kreigman (ed.) *American psychiatry: past, present and future.* Charlottesville: University Press of Virginia.

Ross, A.D. (1961) *The Hindu Family and its Mother–Daughter Bond.* Toronto: University of Toronto Press.

Roth, M. and Kroll, J. (1986) *The Reality of Mental Illness.* Cambridge: Cambridge University Press.

Rothman, D. (1971) *The Discovery of the Asylum.* Boston: Little Brown.

Ruesch, H. (1992) *Naked Empress or the Great Medical Fraud.* Massagne and Lugano: CIVIS Publication.

Runnheim, V.A. (1996) Medicating students with emotional and behavioural disorders and ADHD: a state survey. *Behavioural Disorders* 21: 306–314.

Rutter, M. (1986) Child psychiatry: looking 30 years ahead. *Journal of Child Psychology and Psychiatry* 27: 803–841.

Rutter, M., Graham, P. and Yule, W. (1970a) *A Neuropsychiatric Study of Childhood.* London: Spastics International Medical Publications.

Rutter, M., Tizard, J. and Whitmore, K. (1970b) *Education, Health and Behaviour.* London: Longman.

Rutter, M., Taylor, E. and Hersov, L. (eds) (1994) *Child and Adolescent Psychiatry, Modern Approaches* third edition. Oxford: Blackwell Scientific Publications.

Safer, D.J. and Kraeger, J.M. (1988) A survey of medication treatment for hyperactive inattentive students. *Journal of the American Medical Association* 260: 2256–2258.

Said, H.K. (1983) 'The Unani system of health and medicare' in R.H. Bannerman, J. Burton and L. Wen-Chieh (eds) *Traditional Medicine and Healthcare*. Geneva: World Health Organisation.

Saks, M.J. (1996) The role of research in implementing the UN convention on the rights of the child. *American Psychologist* 51: 1262–1266.

Sandberg, S. (1996) Hyperkinetic or attention deficit disorder. *British Journal of Psychiatry* 169: 10–17.

Sarbin, T. and Kitsuse, J. (eds) (1994) *Constructing the Social*. Thousand Oaks: Sage.

Sartorius, N., Jablensky, A. and Shapiro, R. (1977) Two year follow up of patients included in the WHO international pilot study of schizophrenia. *Psychological Medicine* 7: 529–541.

Sartorius, N. Jablensky, A. and Shapiro, R. (1986) Early manifestation and first contact incidence of schizophrenia *Psychological Medicine* 16: 909–928.

Schachar, R.J. (1991) Childhood hyperactivity. *Journal of Child Psychology and Psychiatry* 32: 155–91.

Schachar, R. and Tannock, R. (1997) Behavioural, situational and temporal effects of treatment of ADHD with methylphenidate. *Journal of the American Academy of Child and Adolescent Psychiatry* 36: 754–763.

Schieffelin, E. (1985) 'The cultural analysis of depressive affect: an example from New Guinea' in A. Kleinman and B. Good (eds) *Culture and Depression*. Berkley: University of California Press.

Schmidt, M.H., Esser, G., Allehoff, W., Geisel, B., Laught, M. and Woerner, W. (1987) Evaluating the significance of minimal brain dysfunction – results of an epidemiological study. *Journal of Child Psychology and Psychiatry* 28: 803–821.

Schmidt, Y., Morozov, G. and Badalyan, L. (1973) 'Letter from the presidium of the All-union Society of Neurologists and Psychiatrists, to the *Guardian*' reprinted in S. Bloch and P. Reddaway (1977) *Russia's Political Hospitals*, London: Victor Gallancz.

Schneider, B.H., Smith, A., Poisson, S.E. and Kwan, A.B. (1997) 'Cultural dimensions of children's peer relations' in S.W. Duck (ed.) *Handbook of Personal Relationships: Theory, Research and Interventions* second edition. Chichester: John Wiley.

Scull, A. (1979) *Museums of Madness*. London: Allen Lane.

Seabrook, J. (1982) *Working Class Childhood: an Oral History*. London: Gollancz.

Shen, Y.C., Wong, Y.F. and Yang, X.L. (1985) An epidemiological investigation of minimal brain dysfunction in six elementary schools in Beijing. *Journal of Child Psychology and Psychiatry* 26: 777–788.

Shotter, J. (1993) *Conversational Realities: Constructing Life through Language*. Thousand Oaks: Sage.

Shweder, R.A. (1991) *Thinking through Cultures: Expeditions in Cultural Psychology*. Cambridge, MA: Harvard University Press.

Shweder, R.A. and Bourne, E.J. (1982) 'Does the concept of the person vary cross-culturally?', in A.J. Marsella and G.M. White (eds) *Cultural Conceptions of Mental Health and Therapy*. Dordrecht: D. Reidel Publishing Company.

Silberg, J., Rutter, M., Meyer, J. *et al.* (1996) Genetic and environmental influences on the covariation between hyperactivity and conduct disturbance in juvenile twins. *Journal of Child Psychology and Psychiatry* 37: 803–816.

Sil-Vestrov, V. (1968) 'Definition of the "disease" concept – the key to discovery of general particular and specific regularities of pathology'. *Archives of Pathology* 30: 90–92.

Simons, R. (1980) The resolution of the Latah paradox. *Journal of Nervous and Mental Disease* 168: 195–206.

Singelis, T.M., Triandis, H.C., Bhawuk, D.S. and Gelfand, M. (1995) Horizontal and vertical dimensions of individualism and collectivism: a theoretical and measurement refinement. *Cross-cultural Research* 29: 240–275.

Sinha, D. (1988) 'The family scenario in a developing country and its implications for mental health: the case of India' in P. Dasen, J. Berry and N. Sartorius (eds) *Health and Cross-cultural Psychology: Towards Applications*. Beverly Hills: Sage.

Sivanandan, A. (1990) *Communities of Resistance – Writings on Black Struggles for Socialism*. London: Verso.

Snezhnevsky, A. (1971) 'The symptomatology, clinical forms and nosology of schizo-phrenia' in J.G. Howels (ed.) *Modern Perspectives in World Psychiatry*. New York: Mazel.

Snezhnevsky, A. and Vartanyan, M. (1970) 'The forms of schizophrenia and their biological correlates' in H. Himwich (ed.) *Biochemistry, Schizophrenia and Affective Illness*. Baltimore: Williams & Wilkins.

Solanto, M.V. and Wender, E.H. (1989) Does methylphenidate constrict cognitive func-tioning? *Journal of the American Academy of Child Adolescent Psychiatry* 28: 897–902.

Solomon, M.F. (1990) Narcissistic vulnerability in marriage. *Journal of Couples Therapy* 1: 25–38.

Sommerville, J. (1982) *The Rise and Fall of Childhood*. London: Sage.

Sonuga-Barke, E.J.S., Minocha, K., Taylor, E.A. and Sandberg, S. (1993) Inter-ethnic bias in teachers ratings of childhood hyperactivity. *British Journal of Developmental Psychology* 11: 187–200.

Sonuga-Barke, E.J.S., Houlberg, K. and Hall, M. (1994) On dysfunction and function in psychological models of childhood disorder. *Journal of Child Psychology and Psychiatry* 35: 1247–1253.

Sow, F. (1985) Muslim families in contemporary Black Africa. *Current Anthropology* 26: 563–573.

Speltz, M.C. (1990) 'The treatment of preschool conduct problems' in M.T. Greenberg, D. Cicchetti, and E.M. Cummings (eds) *Attachment in the Preschool Years*. Chicago: University of Chicago Press.

Spencer, T., Biederman, J., Wilens, T., Harding, M., O'Donnell, D. and Griffin, S. (1996) Pharmacotherapy of attention deficit hyperactivity disorder across the life cycle. *Journal of the American Academy of Child and Adolescent Psychiatry* 35: 409–432.

Sprague, S.L. and Sleator, E.K. (1977) Methylphenidate in hyperkinetic children: differ-ences in dose effects on learning and social behaviour. *Science* 198: 1274–1276.

Stanton, M.E. (1995) 'Patterns of kinship and residence' in B.B. Ingoldsby and S. Smith (eds) *Families in Multicultural Perspective*. New York: Guilford Press.

Steinberg, D. (1994) 'Adolescent services' in M. Rutter, E. Taylor and L. Hersov (eds) *Child and Adolescent Psychiatry, Modern Approaches* third edition. Oxford: Blackwell Scientific Publications.

Steinhausen, H.C. and Erdin, A. (1991) A comparison of ICD-9 and ICD-10 diagnosis of child and adolescent disorders. *Journal of Child Psychology and Psychiatry* 32: 909–920.

Stephens, S. (1995) 'Children and the politics of culture in late capitalism' in S. Stephens (ed.) *Children and the Politics of Culture*. New Jersey: Princeton University Press.

Stevenson, J. and Graham, P. (1988) Behavioural deviances in 13-year-old twins: an item analysis. *Journal of the American Academy of Child and Adolescent Psychiatry* 27: 791–797.

Stewart, M.A., De Blois, S. and Cummings, C. (1980) Psychiatric disorder in the parents of hyperactive boys and those with conduct disorder. *Journal of Child Psychology and Psychiatry* 21: 283–292.

Stiefel, I. (1997) Can disturbance in attachment contribute to attention deficit hyperactivity disorder? A case discussion. *Clinical Child Psychology and Psychiatry* 2: 45–64.

Still, G.F. (1902) Some abnormal psychiatric conditions in children. *Lancet* I: 1008–1012, 1077–1082, 1163–1168.

Strathern, M. (1992) *After Nature: English Kinship in the Late Twentieth Century.* Cambridge: Cambridge University Press.

Strauss, A. and Lehtinen. L. (1947) *Psychopathology and education of the brain-injured child.* New York: Grune & Stratton.

Sullivan, M. (1986) In what sense is contemporary medicine dualistic? *Culture, Medicine and Psychiatry* 10: 331–350.

Szasz, T. (1961) *The Myth of Mental Illness: Foundations of a Theory of Personal conduct.* New York: Hoeber-Harper.

Szasz, T. (1987) *Insanity: the Idea and its Consequences.* New York: Wiley.

Szatmari, P., Offord, D.R. and Boyle, M.H. (1989a) Ontario child health study: prevalence of attention deficit disorder with hyperactivity. *Journal of Child Psychology and Psychiatry* 30: 219–230.

Szatmari, P., Boyle, M. and Offord, D.R. (1989b) ADDH and conduct disorder: degree of diagnostic overlap and differences among correlates. *Journal of the American Academy of Child and Adolescent Psychiatry* 28: 865–872.

Tamasese, K. and Waldegrave, C. (1993) Cultural and gender accountability in the 'Just Therapy' approach. *Journal of Feminist Family Therapy* 5: 29–51.

Tambiah, S.J. (1968) The magical power of words. *Man* 3: 175–208.

Taylor, C. (1985) *Philosophy and the Human Sciences. Philosophical Papers II.* Cambridge: Cambridge University Press.

Taylor, E. (1988) 'Attention deficit and conduct disorder syndromes' in M. Rutter, A.H. Tuma and I.S. Lann (eds) *Assessment and diagnosis in child psychopathology.* New York: Guilford Press.

Taylor, E. (1994) 'Syndromes of attention deficit and overactivity' in M. Rutter, E. Taylor and L. Hersov (eds) *Child and Adolescent Psychiatry, Modern Approaches* third edition. Oxford: Blackwell Scientific Publications.

Taylor, E. and Hemsley, R. (1995) Treating hyperkinetic disorders in childhood. *British Medical Journal* 310: 1617–1618.

Taylor, E. and Werry, J.S. (1994) 'Schizophrenic and allied disorders' in M. Rutter, E. Taylor and L. Hersov (eds) *Child and Adolescent Psychiatry, Modern Approaches* third edition. Oxford: Blackwell Scientific Publications.

Taylor, E., Schachar, R., Thorley, G., Weiselberg, H.M., Everitt, B. and Rutter, M. (1987) Which boys respond to stimulant medication? A controlled trial of methylphenidate in boys with disruptive behaviour. *Psychological Medicine* 17: 121–143.

Taylor, E., Sandberg, S., Thorley, G. and Giles, S. (1991) *The epidemiology of childhood hyperactivity.* Maudsley Monographs No. 33, Oxford: Oxford University Press.

Thapar, A., Hervas, A. and McGuffin, P. (1995) Childhood hyperactivity scores are highly heritable and show sibling competition effects: twin study evidence. *Behavioural Genetics* 25: 537–544.

Timimi, S. (1995) Adolescence in immigrant Arab families. *Psychotherapy* 32: 141–149.

Toone, B. and Van Der Linden, G.J.H. (1997) Attention deficit hyperactivity disorder or hyperkinetic disorder in adults. *British Journal of Psychiatry* 170: 489–491.

Torrey, E.F., Torrey, B.B. and Burton-Bradley, B.G. (1974) The epidemiology of schizo-phrenia in Papua New Guinea. *American Journal of Psychiatry* 131: 567–573.

Trawick, M. (1990) 'The ideology of love in a Tamil family' in O.M. Lynch (ed.) *Divine Passions: the Social Construction of Emotion in India*. Berkley: University of California Press.

Trawick, M. (1991) An Ayurvedic theory of cancer. *Medical Anthropology* 13: 121–136.

Triandis, H.C. (1995) *Individualism and Collectivism*. Boulder, CO: Westview Press.

Trickett, E.J. and Buchanan, R.M. (1997) 'The role of personal relationships in transitions: contributions of an ecological perspective' in S. Duck (ed.) *Handbook of Personal Relationships: Theory, Research and Interventions*. second edition. Chichester: John Wiley.

Tudge, J., Hogan, D., Lee, S. *et al.* (1997) 'Cultural hetero-geneity: parental values and beliefs and their pre schoolers activities in the United States, South Korea, Russia and Estonia' in A. Goncu (ed.) *Children's Engagement in the World*. New York: Cambridge University Press.

Turner, V. (1967) *The Forest of Symbols*. Ithaca, NY: Cornell University Press.

Tyrer, P. (1996) Co-morbidity or consanguinity. *British Journal of Psychiatry* 168: 669–671.

United Nations General Assembly (1989) *Adoption of a convention on the rights of the child*. UN Doc. A/Res/44/25. Nov.1989, New York: United Nations.

United States Department of Education (1991) *Memorandum September 16th: Clarification of Policy to Address the Needs of Children with Attention Deficit Disorders*. Washington, DC: United States Department of Education.

Ujjwalarani, M.V. (1992) Need and scope for counselling psychology in India. *Indian Journal of Behaviour* 16: 8–11.

Van Der Meere, J.J. (1996) 'The role of attention' in S.T. Sandberg (ed.) *Monographs in Child and Adolescent Psychiatry: Hyperactive Disorders of Childhood*. Cambridge: Cambridge University Press.

Van Hoorne, E. (1992) Changes? What changes? The views of the European patients' movement. *International Journal of Social Psychiatry* 38: 30–35.

Van Praag, H.M. (1996) Comorbidity (psycho)analysed. *British Journal of Psychiatry* 168 (Supplement 30): 129–134.

Vergin, N. (1985) Social change and the family in Turkey. *Current Anthropology* 26: 571–574.

Volkow, N.D., Ding, Y.S., Fowler, J.S. *et al.* (1995) Is methylphenidate like cocaine? *Archives of General Psychiatry* 52: 456–463.

Waldegrave, C. (1990) Just therapy. *Dulwich Centre Newsletter* 1: 5–46.

Waldegrave, C. (1997) 'The challenges of culture to psychology and post modern thinking' in M. McGoldrick (ed.) *Re-visioning Family Therapy: Multicultural Systems Theory and Practice*. New York: Guilford Press.

Wallace, A.F. (1959) 'The institutionalization of cathartic and control strategies in Iroquois religious psychotherapy' in M. Opler (ed.) *Culture and Mental Health*. New York: Macmillan.

Walvin, J. (1982) *A Child's World: a Social History of English Childhood 1800–1914*. Harmondsworth: Penguin.

Warnke, G. (1987) *Gadamer: Hermeneutics, Tradition and Reason*. Stanford: Stanford University Press.

Waters and Kraus (2000) *Ritalin Fraud* Online at http://www.ritalinfraud.com.

Watzlawick, P. (1976) *How Real is Real?* New York: Random House.

Watzlawick, P., Weakland, J. and Fisch, R. (1974) *Change: Principles of Pproblem Formation and Problem Resolution*. New York: Norton.

Wedderburn-Tate, C. (1994) The price of going public. *Nursing Management* 1: 18–19.

Weingarten, K. (1998) The small and the ordinary: the daily practice of a postmodern narrative therapy. *Family Process* 37: 3–15.

Weingarten, K. (1994) *The Mother's Voice – Strengthening Intimacy in Families*. New York: Harcourt Brace.

Weingarten, K. (1995) *Cultural Resistance – Challenging Beliefs about Men, Women and Therapy*. New York: Haworth Press.

Weis, G., Kruger, E., Danielson, U. and Elman, M. (1975) Effect of long-term treatment of hyperactive children with methylphenidate. *Canadian Medical Association Journal* 112: 159–165.

Welner, Z., Welner, A., Stewart, M., Palkes, H. and Wish, E. (1977) A controlled study of siblings of hyperactive children. *Journal of Nervous and Mental Disease* 165: 110–117.

Werry, J.S., Elkind, G.S. and Reeves, J.C. (1987a) Attention deficit, conduct oppositional and anxiety disorders in children. III. Laboratory differences. *Journal of Abnormal Child Psychology* 15: 409–428.

Werry, J.S., Reeves, J.C. and Elkind, G.S. (1987b) Attention deficit, conduct oppositional and anxiety disorders in children. 1. A review of research on differentiating characteristics. *Journal of the American Academy of Child and Adolescent Psychiatry* 26: 133–143.

White, G. and Marsella, A. (1982) 'Introduction: cultural conceptions in mental health research and practice' in A. Marsella and G. White (eds) *Cultural Conceptions of Mental Health and Therapy*. Dordrecht: D. Reidel.

White, M. and Epston, D. (1990) *Narrative Means to Therapeutic Ends*. New York: W.W. Norton.

Widener, A.J. (1998) Beyond Ritalin: the importance of therapeutic work with parents and children diagnosed ADD/ADHD. *Journal of Child Psychotherapy* 24: 267–281.

Wolf, R. (1996) *Marriages and Families in a Diverse Society*. New York: HarperCollins.

Wolraich, M., Windgren, S., Stromquist, A., Milich, R., Davis, C. and Watson, D. (1990) Stimulant medication use by primary care physicians in the treatment of attention deficit hyperactivity disorder. *Paediatrics* 86: 95–101.

Wood, H. (1994) *What do Service Users Want from Mental Health Services?* Report to the audit commission, London: HMSO.

Wooldridge, A. (1995) *Measuring the Mind*. Cambridge: Cambridge University Press.

World Health Organization (1973) *The International Pilot Study of Schizophrenia* volume one. Geneva: World Health Organisation.

World Health Organizsation (1979) *Schizophrenia: an International Follow-up Study*. Chichester: Wiley.

World Health Organization (1990) *International Classification of Diseases* tenth edition. Geneva: World Health Organisation.

Xantian, L. (1985) 'The effect of family on the mental health of the Chinese people' in W. Tseng and D. Wu (eds) *Chinese Culture and Mental Health*. New York: Academic Press.

Yang, C.F. (1988) 'Familism and development: an examination of the role of family in contemporary China mainland, Hong Kong and Taiwan' in D. Sinha and H. Kao (eds) *Social Values and Development: Asian Perspectives*. New Delhi: Sage.

Yang, K.S. (1981) Social orientation and individual modernity among Chinese students in Taiwan. *Journal of Social Psychology* 113: 159–170.

Young, A. (1977) Order, analogy and efficacy in Ethiopian medical divination. *Culture, Medicine and Psychiatry* 1: 183–200.

Zachary, G.P. (1997) 'Male order': boys used to be boys, but do some now see boyhood as a malady? *The Wall Street Journal* 2 May.

Zahn, T.P., Rapoport, J.L. and Thompson, C.L. (1980) Autonomic and behavioural effects of dextroamphetamine and placebo in normal and hyperactive pre-pubertal boys. *Journal of Abnormal Child Psychology* 8: 145–160.

Zimmerman, F. (1987) *The Jungle and the Aroma of Meats: an Ecological Theme in Hindu Medicine*. Berkley: University of California Press.

Zwi, M., Ramchandani, P. and Joughlin, C. (2000) Evidence and belief in ADHD. *British Medical Journal* 321: 975–976.

Index

Franklin Pierce College Library

0014161 0